DATE DUE

DEMCO 38-296

Applications Of The Oldest Medicine To The Newest Disease

AIDS

A N D

CHINESE MEDICINE

By Qingcai Zhang, M.D. And Hong-yen Hsu, Ph.D.

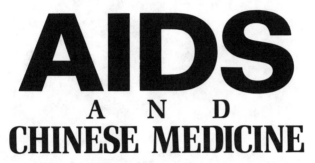

愛滋病之漢方診療

Edited by Heidi Ziolkowski

OHAI PRESS

ORIENTAL HEALING ARTS INSTITUTE
1945 Palo Verde Avenue • Suite 208 • Long Beach,CA 90815

ISBN: 0-941942-31-7

Published by the Oriental Healing Arts Institute
1945 Palo Verde Avenue, Suite 208
Long Beach, California 90815

First Printing: March 1990

Library of Congress Cataloging-in-Publication Data

Zhang, Qingcai, 1938-
    AIDS and Chinese medicine.

    Includes bibliographical references.
    1. AIDS (Disease)—Alternative treatment. 2. Medicine,
Chinese. 3. Herbs—Therapeutic use. I. Hsü, Hung-yüan.
II. Ziolkowski, Heidi. III. Title. [DNLM: 1. Acquired Immuno-
deficiency Syndrome—drug therapy. 2. Drugs, Chinese Herbal—
therapeutic use. 3. Medicine, Chinese Traditional.
WD 308 Z63a]
RC607.A26Z43   1990   616.97′92061′0951   90-7071
ISBN 0-941942-31-7

Contents

Editor's Note Regarding Chinese Medical Terminology

The reader should be aware that certain words and phrases shared by Chinese and Western medicine frequently carry very different meanings. Often, during the course of this book, these terms can only be understood in the context of Chinese medical theory. Examples of such terms include "heart," "lung," "kidney," "spleen," and "blood." Whenever words such as these are not used in their conventional Western sense, the reader should consult the glossary for an understanding of their usage in Chinese medicine.

Other English words are not used in Western medicine, but are very important in Chinese medicine. Such terms as "interior," "exterior," "stagnant," "deficiency," "heat," "fire," "dampness," "wind," and "conformation" are of this type and are, therefore, defined in the glossary.

The third and final class of Chinese medical terminology included in the glossary consists of transliterated terms such as "*yin*," "*yang*," and "*qi*." As foreign words, they are also *italicized* in the text.

Western medical terms are not included in the glossary. If any of these terms are unfamiliar, the reader should consult a reliable medical dictionary.

Acknowledgements

Personal and ongoing contact with our patients with AIDS, ARC, and HIV infections has been our most important and most poignant source of information for the writing of this book. We have learned so very much from these men and women, but by far the most striking lesson has been the one of their courage in the face of death. If there is anything positive we can say about the AIDS epidemic, it is that it has provided a catalyst for change within the practice of medicine. Patients have become a part of the medical team, taking an active and often aggressive role in their own healing. To our patients in San Francisco and Los Angeles, we offer our deepest and most heartfelt thanks.

Our thanks, too, to Sun-Ten pharmaceutical corporation and its generous financial backing, which has allowed us to test the efficacy of treating HIV-infected persons with Traditional Chinese Medicine. Our special thanks are given to Daniel Hsu, who organized the clinical research and without whose help we could not have completed our task. To Dr. Misha Cohen of the San Francisco AIDS Alternative Healing Project, who introduced us to this new field of treating AIDS with Chinese medicine, to Dr. Subhuti Dharmananda, who cofounded the Hong-Yen Project, and to Dr. Mark Katz, who read and critiqued our manuscript, we are profoundly grateful.

Ms. Michelle Honick helped us follow the national progression of the epidemic by continually sending us newspaper clippings and by gleaning books for new material. She also served as our first editor, reading and checking the manuscript twice. Dr. Eleanor R. Long and Ms. Barbara C. Enger, former editors of the Oriental Healing Arts Institute, verified nomenclature and rewrote the first chapter. In the final edits, Ms. Heidi Ziolkowski applied grammatical and stylistic polishes to the manuscript, rewriting many passages, checking the consistency of bibliographic references, writing the glossary and indexing the text. The enormous editorial work of these four women was essential, and we wish to thank all the OHAI staff for their advice and assistance.

Although our research carried with it a calculated risk to our own health and safety, our families did not attempt to dissuade us from continuing our work. Rather, they displayed an empathic understanding for our patients and a selfless realization of the importance of our task. As in all that we do, their emotional support helps us muster our own internal reserves of courage, so that we may fight to the bitter end.

Preface

The basis for Western medicine's focus on specific disease agents may be traced to the publication, in 1858, of Rudolph Virchow's book on cellular pathology. In the decades which followed, Louis Pasteur, Robert Koch and others originated the science of bacteriology, demonstating that many devastating diseases were due to invasion of the body by microscopic parasites. In 1904, German researcher Paul Ehrlich cured an infected animal with a drug which rendered the causal parasite ineffectual, thereby establishing chemical treatment as an approach which is widely practiced to this day.

Due to the empirically-based methods of these pioneers and those of medical scientists of this century, Western medicine has made an incalculable contribution to the betterment of humanity. Most bacterial infections, for instance, are now controlled through inoculation, allowing most people to live longer and healthier lives.

Many diseases, however, remain intractable. Viral infections, metabolic disorders, neoplastic tumors, and genetic dysfunctions elude cures. Since the discovery of a new viral infection, Acquired Immunodeficiency Syndrome (AIDS), in 1981, the deficiencies inherent in the Western approach to healing have become more obvious.

In just eight short years since the discovery of the first verified case, AIDS has spread to more than 157 countries, and the World Health Organization estimates that some ten million people have already been infected with the Human Immunodeficiency Virus (HIV). To date, more than 250,000 full-blown AIDS cases have been diagnosed. In the United States alone, the number of AIDS patients is fast approaching 200,000. The Center for Disease Control estimates that, by 1992, the number of American AIDS patients will reach 365,000. In the next decade, as those 1.5 million Americans already infected with the virus develop AIDS, the entire society will succumb to the tremendous financial and emotional burden of this epidemic, which, if unarrested, could jeopardize the continuance of our species.

Just as some day the ravages of the AIDS virus may incapacitate our global community, it now acts to debilitate the immune systems of infected persons, causing them to become extremely weak and waste away. This stressed condition makes the patient particularly vulnerable to various opportunistic diseases, such as protozoal, fungal, bacterial, and viral infections, and opportunistic cancers.

The United States government's AIDS research budget is the largest in the world, exceeding the combined research budgets for all U.S. government-sponsored cancer and cardiovascular-disease programs. Despite great outlays of time, energy and money, however, the search for a safe antiviral drug or vaccine remains an elusive and frequently frustrating one. Realizing that every day 150 AIDS patients die, we felt the time for action is the present. We decided to join in the efforts to combat AIDS through the application of the techniques and treatments of Traditional Chinese Medicine to this modern-day plague.

The clinical therapeutics of Traditional Chinese Medicine were formulated 1800 years ago by the revered Chinese sage Zhang Zhongjing. His timeworn masterpieces *Shang Han Lun* and *Jin Guei Yao Lue* established TCM diagnostics which are still adhered to by today's TCM practitioners.

First and foremost, TCM emphasizes treatments which enhance the body's natural immunities so that it may more effectively resist disease. Specifically, the fundamental principles of TCM for the treatment of infectious diseases are: *fuzheng* (supporting the body's natural order, i.e. enhancing immunity), and *quxie* (eliminating external evil, i.e. reducing the potency of the pathogen). In this book, the authors expertly summarize the applications of these basic principles to the treatment of AIDS patients.

The touchstone between ancient principals and this modern epidemic is the similarity in the constitutional changes of AIDS patients and the symptom patterns of *xu lao* (asthenia) and *lao zhai* (consumptive exhaustion) described in TCM classics. The enormous amount of literature accumulated over the past 2000 years about *xu sun* (deficiency disorders) has provided a secure theoretical and clinical basis for guiding the treatment of AIDS.

Based on a literature review and clinical practice, the authors designed three groups of herbal formulas:

1. Those antiviral and immuno-enhancing formulas which are directed at the etiological factors and pathogensis of AIDS;

2. Those formulas for non-specific constitutional changes, such as night sweats, low-grade fever, lethargy, and weight loss; and

3. Those formulas designed specifically for opportunistic diseases.

These formulas were devised with both the need to apply treatments to many infected patients with similar symptom patterns (generalization) and the need to administer to the specific conditions of each patient (individualization). In short, to develop effective treatments, a general plan of action was essential, but in clinical practice, catering to the unique complications of each patient was required.

These formulas were the culmination of two years' work into the treatment of AIDS with TCM. In cooperation with the San Francisco AIDS Alternative Healing Project, the Oriental Healing Arts Institute began, in March of 1988, a six-month clinical trial of herbal therapy with AIDS patients. The results of these systematic clinical observations and laboratory tests were reported at the Chinese Medicine Symposium "AIDS, Immunity and Chinese Medicine," sponsored by OHAI in October, 1988 – the first symposium of its kind in the United States. Afterwards, a proceedings of the entire symposium was published by OHAI under the same name. Our work did not stop there, however, as we have continued with clinical observations in the Los Angeles area, and, in October of last year, we had our second symposium on the same topic in an attempt to gain more attention and recognition for this new field. The proceedings will soon be available in book form. In addition to the publication of this book, one of the authors is currently completing a second book on AIDS and Chinese medicine, which should be ready for distribution by the middle of this year. In these ways, we hope to make a contribution to this important task.

The aim of the current book is twofold: (1) to help TCM practitioners understand and use TCM correctly in treating AIDS, and (2) to explain TCM principles and methods of treating AIDS to Western physicians and other health-care providers. Every effort has been made to provide explanations in modern scientific terms. The AIDS patient can also benefit from this work, since it can provide him or her with vital information on alternative means to combatting the virus. This work, however, is not exhaustive. Rather it is meant as an introduction to the use of Traditional Chinese Medicine in the battle against the newest disease. As with all that we publish, we await the comments and suggestions of our readers.

Charleson C. Hsu, Ph.D.
Director, Oriental Healing Arts Institute
Long Beach, California
March 1990

1

Introduction

The Center for Disease Control in Atlanta has predicted that, by 1992, the number of Acquired Immunodeficiency Syndrome (AIDS) cases in the United States will reach 365,000, and that morbidity and mortality rates will increase markedly as the million or more Americans who presently are infected with the Human Immunodeficiency Virus (HIV) progress to the AIDS and AIDS-Related Condition (ARC) stages. (Heyward and Curran 1988). Unofficial sources consider these estimates far too conservative and put their figures as much as three times this high (Masters et al. 1988; Hopkins and Johnston 1988). Of the 105,950 verified AIDS cases reported to the Center for Disease Control as of August 31, 1989, 61,655, or 58% of the total, are no longer living; of those identified before 1985, more than 80% have expired.

Although only 182,463 verified cases had been reported to the World Health Organization as of October 1, 1989, Jonathan M. Mann, director of WHO's Global Program on AIDS, has estimated the actual number to be well in excess of 500,000. Extrapolating from the available data, he believes the total number of HIV (+) individuals to be five million, with one million of those expected to develop AIDS within the next five years. "While it has become fashionable," he cautioned 7000 participants in the Fourth International Conference on AIDS, "to reassure and state that HIV will never threaten certain populations, . . . virology, immunology, social science, and epidemiology require us to take the long view-- and the more somber view" (Mann 1988; WHO 1988; Coulis 1988). The conference, held in Stockholm, Sweden, in June 1988, heard more than 3600 scientific papers, including numerous reports on the proliferation of AIDS throughout the world (Coulis 1988).

To date, no conventional or alternative medicine has been successful in the effort to destroy the AIDS virus or in controlling the damage it causes. No doctor, not even the best informed, can answer all the questions which need to be asked. The individual who has been diagnosed HIV (+), ARC, or AIDS is thus confronted with three possibilities for action:

He or she may choose to trust conventional advice completely, following whatever regimen the doctor in question recommends.

He or she may choose to turn away completely from conventional advice, seeking alternative treatment strategies on the basis of his or her own intuition or judgment.

He or she may choose to explore both conventional and alternative treatment modes with the help of a sympathetic medical practitioner.

It is to this last patient that Traditional Chinese Medicine (TCM) offers a sensible, practical, and responsible approach. It has long been recognized that persons who are active participants in their own therapeutic process fare much better than those who play only a passive role (Siegel 1986). Because Traditional Chinese Medicine emphasizes the well-being of the whole person, not the targeting of isolated pathologies, it encourages the patient to cooperate or even take the initiative in identifying problems and developing the overall strategies which will be of greatest benefit for the solution of these problems.

This book is addressed first of all, then, to persons who have been diagnosed with AIDS or ARC and who are seeking forms of treatment which can help them in their struggle to stay alive and functional. To such persons, Traditional Chinese Medicine offers an integrated system of herbal therapy, acupuncture, moxibustion, manipulation, and breathing exercises, a holistic approach which serves to balance and strengthen the body so that the body can heal itself.

Although the potential role of Traditional Chinese Medicine in healing AIDS and ARC has been recognized by some advocates of natural therapies (Badgley 1986; O'Connor 1986, 1987), no previous attempt has been made to present, in a concrete and systematic fashion, the ways in which TCM may be able to benefit sufferers from acquired immune-deficiency syndromes. For example, experience with immune-system deficiency resulting from chemotherapy or radiotherapy treatment, both in cancer and in organ-transplant cases, has demonstrated the efficacy of TCM in counteracting the immune-suppressing effects of such treatments (Andrews 1987; Dong 1978; Hanbing Huang et al. 1982; Jiang et al. 1979; Liao et al. 1982; Jiaqing Zhang et al. 1987; Lou et al. 1983; Sun Yan et al. 1987). It is therefore reasonable to hope that the virally-introduced acquired immune-deficiency syndromes known as AIDS and ARC will respond in a similar fashion, at least in some cases.

Because of its emphasis on preventive treatment, Traditional Chinese Medicine also offers a practical methodology for persons who, while still enjoying fairly good health, have tested positive for AIDS virus antibodies (HIV+) and thus live under constant threat of invasion by opportunistic diseases. In ancient Chinese medical tenets, the highest praise was accorded to practitioners who treated their patients while they were healthy, rather than waiting for substantial pathological damage to occur. The superior physician, it was held, was one whose diagnoses and treatments prevented disease, not one who merely cured the disease after it had developed (Wong and Wu 1925). The techniques for maintaining sound health and forestalling disease which were developed in accordance with this principle are particularly appropriate to the HIV (+) condition, enabling the affected individual to marshal his own body's resources against the expected attack.

It follows that all health care professionals who may be called upon to care for AIDS/ARC and HIV(+) persons can profit from an understanding of the principles of Traditional Chinese Medicine which this book endeavors to provide. The allopathic approach of conventional Western medicine, valuable though it is, is vulnerable to the development of drug-resistant germs and viruses as well as to the accompaniment of unwelcome side effects. In such complicated epidemic diseases as AIDS/ARC, its one-disease-one-cause-one-cure approach may fall somewhat short of an optimal course of treatment. In contrast, Traditional Chinese Medicine has always paid primary attention to the patient's entire body, seeing pathogens as external factors of secondary importance rather than the specific or exclusive targets of therapy. Even if we assume that modern medical research can find the "magic bullet" which will eradicate the AIDS virus, the profound pathogenic alterations it has created in the invaded body will remain a problem which, from the point of view of TCM, is a far more important consideration than is its etiology. A badly ruined body needs to be "rebuilt," and TCM offers both the theoretical basis and the tested procedures for doing so.

Finally, the rapid spread of the AIDS/ARC epidemic will inevitably bring many of these AIDS/ARC and HIV(+) patients to practitioners of Traditional Chinese Medicine seeking relief through acupuncture treatment and/or herbal therapy. Indeed, a number of TCM physicians have been treating AIDS and ARC patients experimentally for several years, using a variety of TCM approaches, including acupuncture, moxibustion, breathing exercises, and herbal formulas (Misha Cohen 1986, 1987, 1988; Smith 1987; Barton 1988; Dharmananda 1987, 1988). Their pioneering work will be described in full in a subsequent chapter, together with a discussion of the therapeutic principles involved. It should be immediately apparent, however, that practitioners of Traditional Chinese Medicine need to be as fully informed as possible about AIDS, its origin and nature, and its symptoms, so that they may be adequately prepared to care for patients seeking their help.

Even among conventional Western medical practitioners, such information is frequently lacking. A recent survey of 1000 general practitioners and internists in the state of California indicated that only 16-20% of them were familiar enough with AIDS symptomatology to diagnose the condition, and only 35% routinely inquired about their patients' sexual behavior

(Clark 1986, 1987). This is not at all surprising. Few of the physicians practicing today, either in conventional Western medicine or in TCM, were (or could have been) taught to recognize and treat AIDS victims, nor were they likely to have been made sufficiently aware of contributing social factors, such as the diverse sexual habits and the pervasiveness of drug abuse which have made the spread of AIDS possible.

Recognizing the overwhelming threat presented by the AIDS virus, as well as the demonstrated value of a therapeutic procedure which combines Western medical technology with Chinese medicine, this book is intended to serve patients, Western practitioners, and TCM practitioners as a useful source of information which will enable all three to work together. For example, the diagnosis of AIDS/ARC or HIV (+) is best arrived at by a conventional Western doctor. When Western drug therapies are utilized, their side effects can be minimized by herbal formulas prescribed by a TCM practitioner, and using TCM procedures, the patient can help himself to strengthen his body's resistance to disease.

Traditional Chinese Medicine is a complete organized medical system, the second largest in the world. It is not to be confused with folk medicine or with hucksterism; its theories are of ancient provenance, and in clinical practice today it serves over a billion people. In China, Japan, and Southeast Asia, it is recognized as an official medical component to be integrated with, not supplanted by, the practice of Western medicine. Such an integrated policy was adopted by the People's Republic of China in 1949 and by the Japanese government in 1976.

The AIDS information presented here is derived both from published literature and from clinical experiments conducted by the San Francisco AIDS Alternative Healing Project in collaboration with the Oriental Healing Arts Institute and Brion Herbs Corporation. Publication of this information, however, entails no categorical assurance of its reliability. AIDS research is still in the experimental stage, and its implications, as reported both here and elsewhere, must be understood in that light by concerned AIDS sufferers and their physicians.

2

Oldest Medicine,
Brand-New Disease

Acquired Immunodeficiency Syndrome (AIDS) is the Western disease name for a contagious disease, caused by a viral infection, that was first identified only eight years ago. The pathogenic virus is now called Human Immunodeficiency Virus (HIV); names used previously were Human T-cell Lymphotropic Virus Type III (HTLV-III), Lymphadenopathy-Associated Virus (LAV), and AIDS-associated Retrovirus (ARV). It is a highly mutable virus, a large number of variants of which have already been discovered.

Acquired means that the disease comes from contact with someone or something carrying the AIDS virus (HIV). So far as is known, however, the only modes of contact through which HIV may be transmitted from one person to another are those involving a literal exchange of specific bodily fluids, i.e. sexual intercourse, blood transfusions, and the mingling of infected blood with that of the recipient, either through accidental wounding or, more commonly, through the sharing of needles in the practice of intravenous drug use.

Immunodeficiency means that the essence of the disease is the infected body's loss of its natural immunity, so that it cannot resist further infection by destroying or expelling the invading organisms. While immunodeficiency may be acquired, as in HIV infections, it may also be induced by medications used to suppress immune-system rejection in patients undergoing organ transplants or chemo- or radiotherapy for the treatment of cancer.

Syndrome means that the AIDS is not a single distinctive entity but a loose pattern of objective signs and subjective symptoms, depending on the nature of the opportunistic infection which the HIV infection has rendered the body powerless to resist. Such viral infection as herpes, EBV and CMV are common, as are fungal infections like candidiasis, mycobacterial infections like tuberculosis, and protozoal infections like *Pneumocystis carinii* pneumonia. Other possible symptoms include swollen lymph glands, the neoplastic lesion known as Kaposi's sarcoma, fever, night sweating, chest rales, diarrhea, weight loss, and acute and chronic fatigue.

Immunodeficiency is not in itself fatal to the body's vital system. However, the opportunistic diseases noted above as characteristic manifestations of AIDS do not normally occur, or at the very least, do not become life-threatening, in persons with intact immune systems. It is only when the immune system is ravaged by HIV that such infections are able to invade the body without hindrance, resulting eventually in the death of the victim.

In Traditional Chinese Medicine, exterior pathogenic factors, such as viruses and bacterial and fungal infections, are called "exterior evils." The term is entirely conceptual, deriving as it does from a time when microscopic and other laboratory technology was unknown and the physician was forced to rely entirely upon clinical observation. On this basis, he determined whether the exterior evil responsible for the patient's symptoms represented wind, cold, heat, dampness, dryness, or fire. (Please consult the glossary for TCM definitions of these terms.)

Traditional Chinese Medicine views the body's natural immunity as a function of the individual's vital energy, or *zheng qi* (正氣), and reasons that when an external evil attacks successfully, there must be a deficiency of *zheng qi*. This view corresponds very well to modern theory concerning the invasion of the immunodeficient body by opportunistic disease.

The syndrome or pattern of symptoms in TCM diagnostic terminology is called *zheng* (證), or conformation. Determining the patient's *zheng* begins with an analysis of his symptoms in accordance with the principles of the "four examinations": *wang zhen* (望診) (visual observation), *wen zhen* (聞診) (aural and olfactory observation), *wen zhen* (問診) (questioning diagnosis), and *qie zhen* (palpation). The location, nature, and probable cause of the patient's condition, together with his or her response to treatment, are all taken into account. But conformation is not to be confused with disease; it is rather a total picture of the patient's physiological, mental, and emotional states. Since AIDS is not, properly speaking, a disease entity, the *zheng* concept of diagnosis would seem to be particularly appropriate to treating it, since its clinical manifestations correspond in most cases to the TCM conformation of *xu lao* (虛勞) (asthenic disease), in advanced cases to the TCM conformation of *lao zhai* (勞瘵) (consumptive exhaustion).

Since, etiologically, AIDS is a viral infection, pathophysiologically, AIDS damages the immune system of the body, and, clinically, it shows mostly deficient symptoms. To apply Traditional Chinese Medicine to the AIDS treatment, we should first examine how TCM deals with viral diseases, immunity, and deficiencies.

Traditional Chinese Medicine and Viral Infections

In ancient times, Chinese people called the epidemic diseases *yi* (疫), *wenyi* (瘟疫), *yili* (疫癘), and *shiyi* (時疫). These diseases were recorded in the earlest Chinese written language of the inscriptions on bones and tortoise shells of Yin dynasty (16th to 11th century B.C.). There were more than 100 Chinese characters describing the epidemic diseases on these bones and shells. *Huang-di Nei-jing* (Inner Classic of the Yellow Emperor, written around 100 B.C.) described the epidemic diseases as "the occurrance of five pestilences (a general term for all kinds of epidemic diseases) which are transmitted among the people. The symptoms are similar, no matter at what age." Prevention was emphasized in this classic work. It advised physicians to treat persons before they were attacked by a disease.

During the East Han dynasty (25-220 A.D.), there were numerous epidemic diseases, then termed *shan han* (febrile diseases). A full two-thirds of the members of the Zhang Zhong-jing family died from these diseases, which stimulated the patriarch to summarize the medical literature up to his time. He compiled the first and most influential book on Chinese medical history, *Shan Han Lun* (Treatise on Febrile Diseases), in 217 A.D. Because of Zhang Zhong-jing's seminal work, progress in the recognition, differentiation, and treatment of infectious diseases has been possible. *Zhou-hou Bei-ji Fang* (Emergency Prescriptions to Keep Up One's Sleeve, 341 A.D.) by Ge Hong of the Jin (晉) dynasty (265-419 A.D.), *Zhu-bing Yuan-hou Lun* (Discussion on the Origins of Symptoms in Illness, 610 A.D.) by Chao Yuan-fang, and *Wai-tai Bi-yao* (Necessities of a Frontier Official, 752 A.D.) by

Wang Tao of the Tang dynasty (618-907 A.D.) all have sections on epidemic diseases.

Special monographs on epidemic diseases first appeared during the Ming dynasty (1368-1644 A.D.). By that time, institutes for the study of febrile diseases, as well as eruptive and pustulant diseases, such as smallpox and measles, had been established (Wong and Wu 1977, p. 133). The epidemic diseases such as the poxes and rashes, which we now know mostly as viral diseases, were treated by specialists from the Department of Poxes and Rashes. *Dou-zhen Xin-fa* (Secret Methods for Poxes and Rashes, 1564 A.D.) by Wan Quan may have been the first book specially devoted to those viral diseases in Chinese medical history. It detailed the manifestations of poxes and rashes, including differential diagnosis patterns and their treatments. *Wen-yi Lun* (Discussion of Warm Epidemics, 1642 A.D.) by Wu You-Ke is a preliminary discussion of warm diseases, their mode of infection, their progression in the body, and their prognosis and treatments. Wu You-Ke's book prompted the establishment of a new school in infectious diseases, which were called *wen bing*.

In Wu's *Wen-yi Lun*, the pathogenic factors are called *li qi* (癘氣) (infectious evil factors). This is the first time Wu recognized that there might be another causal contributor other than abnormal weather or external physical factors such as wind, cold, heat, fire, dampness, and dryness. His description of the features of *li qi* had some similarities with the microbiological pathogens we now know. First, he noticed there were different *li qi* which caused different diseases. Second, he noticed that different *li qi* can selectively invade different parts of the body and cause diseases of special organs and meridians. Third, he noticed different levels of susceptibility and immunity among household animals and human beings. Certain *li qi* causes ox illness, but not goat, just as certain *li qi* causes sickness in humans but not in animals. He recognized the varying interactions between different forms of *li qi* with human beings and animals. Later, in the Qing dynasty (1644-1911 A.D.), Ye Tian-shi's *Wen-re Lun* (Discussion of Warm Diseases, 1746 A.D.) and Wu Ju-tong's *Wen-bing Tiao-bian* (Refined Diagnosis of Warm Diseases, 1798 A.D.) discussed the patterns, course, anatomical locations, treatment principles, and herbal formulas for febrile and warm diseases.

In those works, what is now known as influenza is recorded as *feng wen* (wind-warm syndrome) or *dong wen* (winter-warm syndrome). Epidemic encephalitis is recognizable in the descriptions of *shu wen* (summer heat-warm disease) and *fu wen* (seasonal evil-heat disease). Chronic and acute forms of hepatitis were distinguished as *huang dan* (jaundice) and *je huang* (acute jaundice), respectively. Among the warm diseases, *wen tu* (violent evil-heat disease) includes *da tou wen* or mumps. In their discussions of the etiology, diagnosis, and treatment of these so-called "warm" ailments, early practitioners of Traditional Chinese Medicine clearly recognized the infectious nature and presence of external evils, which we now perceive as viruses.

Although modern science has revealed the nature of viral diseases in great detail, we still lack effective therapeutic measures to combat viral infections. This is especially true of chronic viral infections, such as chronic hepatitis B and the Epstein-Barr virus (EBV). Even the most common illnesses, like the flu and colds, we still cannot effectively treat. For the most part, these viral diseases are healed by our body's own natural healing abilities. Since the integration of Western and Chinese traditional medicine, the therapeutic results for certain viral diseases has been greatly improved. In China, these viral diseases have been treated by classic herbal formulas developed thousands of years ago, and also with new formulas which were formulated according to the results of new pharmacological research.

Combined with modern pathological and pharmacological knowledge, TCM has developed systematic therapeutic methods for various viral infections. For example, the Lonicera and Forsythia Formula, prepared by Wu Ju-tong during the Qing dynasty about 300 years ago, has proved quite effective in treating influenza. The formula not only relieves symptoms but actually terminates the disease. A widely-used cure for mumps is the Three Flower Combination, which consists of viola, lonicera, chrysanthamum, and licorice. We will now discuss some of the common viral infections associated with AIDS epidemic in order to illustrate TCM principles for treating virus diseases.

The incidence rate of hepatitis B is very high in the Chinese population. Since there are no effective anti-hepatitis virus drugs available in conventional Western medicine, therapeutic means for treating this disease in China are relegated to TCM. TCM treatments for hepatitis B are focused on removing predisposing factors (e.g. abnormal immunity), inhibiting hepatic degeneration, necrosis and inflammation, promoting hepatic regeneration, inhibiting hyperplasia of collagen, and promoting collagenolysis. There are many herbs that promote the reparation of injured hepatocytes and the regeneration of the necrotic cells. According to various clinical studies, the most efficacious herbs are schizandra, cucumis, salvia, peony, silybum, astragalus and *tang-kuei*. The most effective herbal formulas are Capillaris Combination and *Tang-kuei* and Bupleurum Formula (Han et al. 1988; Song 1987). Ma et al. have combined the TCM differentiation with autonomic functions to increase the therapeutic results of chronic persistent viral hepatitis and obtained a remission rate of 76% (Ma 1988). Hepatitis, as a complication in AIDS/ARC patients, has a noteworthy incidence rate, as the majority of these patients contract the hepatitis B virus at some point during the course of their HIV infestation. The TCM method for treating hepatitis, therefore, has important applications for these patients.

Herpes is another very common complication in AIDS/ARC patients. TCM considers it the dampness-heat blend of the lower energizer. There were several reports on treating herpes with TCM methods. Li Lin et al. of the Chinese Academy of TCM reported that, in 100 patients with herpes zoster treated with *Machixian Jiedu* Decoction, 86 were cured, 10 were markedly improved, and 4 cases were significantly improved. Fifty-three patients were cured in seven days, and 33 were cured in 8-14 days (Li Lin et al. 1985). The ingredients of this treatment are *Portulaca oleracea, Isatis tinctoria, Lithospermum erythrorhizon, Patrinia villosa, Coptis chinensis, Zizyphus spinosa*, and oyster shell. Zemin Zheng et al. reported that 51 cases of herpes zoster were diagosed and differentially treated with TCM. Patients with strong fire in liver and gallbladder conformation were treated with modified Gentiana Combination (see HY-21 in Appendix 3); patients with dampness-heat in spleen and stomach were treated with modified Magnolia and Hoelen Combination; patients with poor flow of vital energy and blood stasis were treated with modified *Tang-kuei* Four Combination (see HY-24 in Appendix 3). All patients were cured, with an average duration of treatment of six days (Zemin Zheng et al. 1984).

Traditional Chinese Medicine and Immunity

Although the term *mian yi*, meaning "immunity" in the sense understood by Western medicine, did not appear in Chinese medical treatises until the publication of *Mian Yi Lei Fang* (Formulas for Conferring Immunity) in the late 19th century, the concept was evident as early as the Tang dynasty (619-907 A.D.), during which Wang Ping published his edition of *Huang Ti Nei Jing Su Wen* (The Yellow Emperor's Classic of Internal Medicine, Simple Questions). A much-cited passage from that work reads as follows: "If you don't want to be contaminated by epidemic disease, *zheng qi* must be integrated into the body; then the external evil cannot invade the body."

Zheng qi (vital energy) is the way in which Traditional Chinese Medicine defines the human body's natural ability to resist disease. One aspect of *zheng qi* is called *wei qi* (defense *qi*); it belongs to the body's *yang* principle, and circulates in superficial parts of the body protecting the integument against external pathogenic evils. The primordial principle is considered to be concerned with *pi qi* (spleen *qi*), the post-natal source of vital *qi*, and *shen qi* (kidney *qi*), the congenital source of vital *qi*. Controlling the circulation of *wei qi* is *fei qi* (lung *qi*). Immunity is thus seen as the function of the three organs--kidney, spleen, and lung--working harmoniously to keep external evils at bay. (For the specialized TCM definitions of these and other organs, please consult the glossary.)

But artificial immunization was also reported during the Tang dynasty. According to Dong Yu-shan's *Niu Tou Xin Shu* (New Treatise on Bovine Diseases):

> There was no such thing as vaccination in ancient times. It was first performed in the early period of the Tang dynasty

in the southern part of the Yangzte River, where Chao first invented a nasal bovine vaccination against smallpox.

This method became popular in China during the 16th century and was taken up in the West in the 17th. Similar procedures have been recorded in the literature of Traditional Chinese Medicine as preventatives against rabies and measles (Meifang Chen 1989).

TCM has developed a system of therapy based on centuries-old empirical observation to deal with immune system deficits. Recently, the efficacy of these Chinese herbal formulas for treating immune deficiencies have been verified by the collaborating work between TCM practitioners and scientific researchers. In an effort to lend scientific credence to their medical knowledge, the Chinese have begun to apply accepted scientific research techniques. The results have been very encouraging. Many investigations have been completed on the effectiveness of Chinese herbs and immunity. Herbs used in China for immunomodulation fall into three general categories: those which enhance the immune system; those which inhibit the immune system; and those which have a nonspecific adaptogenic effect (Halstead 1989). (For detailed information on the immunomodulating effects of Chinese herbs, please see Chapter Seven.)

Investigation of the essence of the *zheng*, or conformation, is to provide the objective pathophysiological evidence and to describe the clinical manifestations in modern scientific terms. This kind of research has been focused on *xu zheng* (asthenic or deficiency illnesses) and their immunodeficiency nature. It seems that to treat AIDS with the principles of treatment for *xu zheng* of TCM is correct. In the last part of this chapter, the data of this kind of research will be discussed.

Traditional Chinese Medicine and AIDS-Like Syndrome

Although AIDS as a disease entity does not occur in the historical literature, the fact that it presents itself as a constellation of varying symptoms renders it especially appropriate for diagnosis and treatment by Traditional Chinese Medicine, which evaluates all disease on the basis of the patient's clinical symptoms and the patterns of those symptoms. The TCM view is that, though the nature of the disease is a basic concern, often treatment can only based on the clinical appearance and the pathophysiological tendency of the disease. This treatment principle, known as "treating different diseases with the same method," has been modified in recent times as Western diagnostic tools have become available and efforts made to reconcile and integrate the two disciplines. Nevertheless, the *zheng*-differentiation approach remains a useful ally in the search for practical methods of coping with AIDS. This is the reason why we are citing the ancient literature on AIDS-like syndromes here and why we can use TCM to treat AIDS.

As was mentioned earlier in the chapter, two *zheng*, or conformations, recognized in the classical literature of Traditional Chinese Medicine very closely resemble the symptoms most frequently manifested in those who have tested positive for the AIDS virus (*xu lao*, asthenic disease), as well as those suffering from AIDS (*lao zhai*, consumptive exhaustion). In *Huang Ti Nei Jing*, these symptoms are identified as deficiencies of *yin, yang, qi, xue, ying, wei,* and the five organs, and are attributed to the collapse of *jing* (essence), *qi* (vital energy), *yie* (bodily fluids) or *xue* (blood). *Huang Ti Nei Jing* attributes such conditions to sexual intemperance, alcohol use and poor hygiene.

Jin Kui Yao Lue (Prescriptions from the Golden Chamber), published in 220 A.D. by Zhang Zhong-jing, is more specific. It describes *xu lao* as either a general debility or a consumptive ailment, caused by impairment of *zang* (the five solid organs) and deficiency of primordial *zheng qi*, including the following variants (Hsu et al. 1983):

- (in men) A pale complexion, excessive thirst, shortness of breath, cardiac palpitation, and a floating pulse are signs of internal weakness, particularly an asthenic condition of *xue* (blood).

- (in men) A pale complexion; shortness of breath; mild chills and fever; dizziness; lower abdominal distention with a sensation of urgent tension; oliguria; and an empty, submerged, and chordal pulse are manifestations of *xu lao*.

- (in men) Aching and emaciated feet which inhibit walking, fever in palms and soles, spermatorrhea and sensation of chill in the pubic area, and a floating and large pulse are signs that the *xu lao* condition is caused by excessive alcohol consumption.

- (in men and women) Shortness of breath when walking; a chilling sensation in the hands and feet; abdominal distention; diarrhea; and a submerged, thin, and slow pulse characterize the condition known as *tao qi*, collapse of *qi*.

Jin Kui Yao Lue also offers prescriptions tailored to the symptomatic patterns displayed by individual patients, as follows.

- (in men) Spermatorrhea may be accompanied by dizziness, hair loss, a tense and urgent sensation in the lower abdomen, a sensation of chilling in the penis, and an extremely weak, hollow and slow pulse; alternatively, a hollow, fluttering, minute and tense pulse may be found. In either case, deficiency of *xue* is to be suspected, and Cinnamon and Dragon Bone Combination is the prescription of choice.

- *Xu lao* with internal cramps and variable deficiencies is usually treated with Astragalus Combination.

- *Xu lao* with lower back pain, cramping in the lower abdomen, and oliguria is treated with Rehmannia Eight Formula.

- *Xu lao* which renders the patient susceptible to wind and *qi* diseases, should be treated with Dioscorea and Jujube Formula.

- *Xu lao* accompanied by insomnia and irritability is treated with *Zizyphus* Combination.

- *Xu lao* featuring internal cramps, cardiac palpitation, nosebleed, soreness and aching of the limbs, fever in palms and soles, dry throat and mouth, and (in men) nocturnal emission may be treated with Minor Cinnamon and Peony Combination.

- *Xu lao* characterized by extreme weakness and anorexia to the point of emaciation, abdominal distention, coarse and scaly skin, and bruising about the eyes is symptomatic of injury to *qi* in the meridians, skin, and internal organs caused by excessive indulgence in food, alcohol, and sex, and by worry and overexertion. Rhubarb and *Eupolyphaga* Formula is recommended.

- Moribund *xu lao*, in which the dying patient manifests extreme fatigue, multiple deficiencies, cardiac palpitation, excessive perspiration, extreme mental depression, and a knotty pulse, should be treated with Baked Licorice Combination.

During the Sui dynasty, Chao Yuan-fang's *Zhu Ping Yuan Hou Lun* (Treatise on the Origins of the Symptoms of All Diseases), published in 610 A.D., classified *xu lao* conditions as *wu lao* (five asthenic diseases), *lu jie* (six exhaustions), and *qi shang* (seven impairments). His work was followed, in 652 A.D., during the Tang dynasty, by Sun Si-mo's *Qian Jin Yao Fang* (Precious Prescriptions) and during the Jin dynasty, in 1174 A.D., by Chen Yen's *San Yin Ji Yi Bing Zheng Fang Lun* (Three Categories of Pathogenic Factors and Symptoms), both of which also discussed the etiology, pathogenesis, and treatment of *xu lao*.

Theories and treatment methods for *xu lao* and *lao zhai* became more sophisticated and mature with the advent of the Yuan dynasty (1206-1368 A.D.). In *Pi Wei Lun* (A Treatise on the Spleen and Stomach), Li Dong-yuan advanced, in 1249 A.D., the theory that *xu lao* is the result of impairment of the spleen and stomach by improper and unbalanced food intake, injury from exterior (weather) evils of hot and cold, and internal impairment of *yuan qi* (original energy) by excess of excitement, worry, or anger. To counteract these evils, he designed a formula known and used today as Ginseng and Astragalus Combination. One hundred years later, in 1347 A.D., Zhu Dan-xi's *Dan Xi Xin Fa* (Dan-xi's Logical Diagnoses) discussed *xu lao* as an aspect of *lao zhai*. His analysis differed from Li Dong-yuan's. On the principle of nourishing *yin* and moderating evil fire, he recommended tonifying kidney by the administration of *Tang-kuei* Four Combination, augmented with *Anemone raddeana* and *Phellodendron amurense* or *da bu yin wan*, Great Universal *Yin* Formula.

The works of these two men inspired competing schools that deeply influenced later developments. The first emphasized the nourishment of spleen and *qi*, while the second, the nourishment of kidney and *yin*.

The major contribution of the Ming dynasty (1368-1644 A.D.) to theoretical and therapeutic insight concerning *xu lao* and *lao zhai* was Zhang Jing-yue's *Jing Yue Quan Shu* (The Complete Works of Jing Yue), published in 1624 A.D. Its comprehensive discussion of etiology, pathogenesis, and treatment classifies the manifestation of *xu lao* as five *lao* (asthenic diseases), *lu ji* (six exhaustions) and *qi shang* (seven impairments), with *lao zhai* representing the extreme condition of *xu lao* (Xianming Wang 1984). The manifestations represent the entire spectrum of asthenic disease and are remarkably comparable to the symptoms experienced by persons with AIDS (PWAs).

The Five *Lao*

These five asthenic organ diseases are the manifestations of *xu lao* in the five visceral systems: *xin lao* (heart asthenia), *gan lao* (liver asthenia), *pi lao* (spleen asthenia), *fei lao* (lung asthenia), and *shen lao* (kidney asthenia). The impairment of *qi* in any of the respective organs brings about malnourishment of the whole visceral system, resulting in pathogenic changes in skin, muscles, blood vessels, tendons, and bones. When such an extreme malfunction of all body systems exists, it is of the greatest importance that differential diagnosis be employed to determine which organ is impaired and whether *qi* or blood is insufficient. Only then can a proper treatment principle and formulas appropriate to the condition be arrived at.

* *Xin Lao* (Heart Asthenia)

Since the heart controls blood vessels, asthenic changes in the heart cause such symptoms as pallid complexion and palpitations. The heart also houses the mind in TCM theory; therefore, heart impairment results in anxiety, fearfulness, dream-disturbed sleep, and insomnia.

* *Gan Lao* (Liver Asthenia)

Mental excitement can damage liver *qi*, producing not only anxiety, but also blurred vision, flaccid muscles and tendons, difficulty of movement, and pain in the chest and hypochondrium.

* *Pi Lao* (Spleen Asthenia)

Overeating and/or excessive worrying damages spleen *qi*. The symptoms of such damage are muscular wasting and weakness in the limbs, abdominal distention, loss of appetite, and loose stool and/or diarrhea.

* *Fei Lao* (Lung Asthenia)

Damage to lung *qi* is indicated by a cough, shortness of breath, sensation of fullness in the chest, back pain, facial emaciation, aversion to chill, and general lassitude.

* *Shen Lao* (Kidney Asthenia)

Kidney *qi* is damaged by excessive sexual activity. Its symptoms include *gu zheng lao re* (debilitating heat steaming from the bones), night sweating, tidal fevers, lumbago and weakness in the lower limbs, as well as spermatorrhea in men and menstrual dysfunction in women.

Lu Ji, The Six Exhaustions

Exhaustion (*ji*) is a complex of deficiency symptoms manifested in *xue* (blood), *qi* (vital energy), *jing* (vital essence), *jin* (tendons), *rou* (muscles), and *gu* (bones).

* *Xue Ji* (Blood Exhaustion)

Two characteristics of blood exhaustion are alopecia and memory loss.

* *Qi Ji* (Exhaustion of Vital Energy)

An obvious indication that *qi* (vital energy) has become depleted is difficulty in breathing: shallow breathing, rapid breathing, or shortness of breath.

* *Jing Ji* (Exhaustion of Vital Essence)

When *jing* (vital essence) becomes exhausted, eye and ear deficiencies, notably blurring of vision and impairment of hearing, are evidenced.

* *Jin Ji* (Tendon Exhaustion)

Exhausted tendons produce muscle spasms and convulsions.

* *Rou Ji* (Muscle Exhaustion)

Degenerated and atrophied muscles are said to be exhausted.

* *Gu Ji* (Bone Exhaustion)

Bone exhaustion reveals itself in loss of teeth and debility in the feet.

Because diseases of the five solid organs interact with each other, it is important to diagnose and cure the disease of any one of them before it affects the others. If most or all of the organs are already affected, treatment becomes extremely difficult. For example, since *pi* (spleen) is the postnatal source of *qi* (vital energy), a disease originating in *fei* (lung) and *shen* (kidney) must be arrested before *pi* is involved, or the resulting destruction of *qi* will render the disease incurable. Similarly *xu lao* (asthenia) will develop into *ji* (exhaustion) unless proper measures based upon the Theory of the Five Solid Organs are implemented.

The Seven *Shang*

Also contributing to the disease conditions encompassed in *xu lao* are the seven impairments, or internal and external causes of undue stress.

*Overeating impairs *pi* (spleen).

*Excessive anger impairs *gan* (liver).

*Overworking and prolonged sitting at a damp place impairs *shen* (kidney).

*Exposure to cold-evil and retenion of water impairs *fei* (lung).

*Worry and anxiety impair *xin* (heart).

*Exposure to wind, rain, cold, and summer-heat evils impairs the constitution.

*Great shock and intemperance impair the mind.

Yin and *Yang* Deficiencies in *Xu Lao*

Manifestations of asthenia, exhaustion, and impairment culminate in deficiency of either *yin* or *yang*; both are common syndromes in *xu lao* disease.

- *Yin* deficiency, in its extreme form, means that the condition exists in all five organs. The symptoms, therefore, are very complicated. The most characteristic are *gu zheng lao re* (debilitating heat steaming from the bones), a sensation of chill, cough, shortness of breath, loss of appetite, anxiety, a sensation of fatigue, hot sensation in palms and soles, and insomnia.

● *Yang* deficiency, again in its extreme form, is always accompanied by *qi* deficiency. Symptoms in this case are
a sensation of heat on the surface of the body, oc-
casional sensation of chill, wheezing upon slight exertion, shortness of breath, sore and aching body, cold
extremities, spontaneous perspiration, anxiety, and
sensation of fatigue.

Lao Zhai (Consumptive Exhaustion)

Consumptive exhaustion is a chronic degenerative condition, the extreme form of *xu lao* (asthenic disease), and is infectious in nature. Its etiology, pathogenesis, and clinical
manifestations, as presented in the classical literature, so closely resemble those of AIDS in its fully-developed stage that it is
appropriate to cite them here.

Both *Qian Jin Yao Fang* (see above) and *Wai Tai Mi Yao*
(Unofficial Medical Secrets), composed by Wang Tao in 752
A.D., described *lao zhai* in detail, emphasizing its infectious
and consumptive nature and warning that failure to understand the proper treatment would result in the extinction of
the "tribe." *San Yin Ji Yi Bing Zheng Fan Lun* (see above) and
Ji-sheng Fang (Life-Preserving Prescriptions), compiled by Yen
Yong He in 1253 A.D., give detailed symptom patterns for 24
clinical sub-types of *lao zhai*. The fourteenth-century *Dan Xi
Xin Fa* (see above) argued that *lao zhai* results from injury to
the physical body and its *qi* (vital energy) through impairment
of *xin* (heart) and *shen* (kidney) by fatigue. Li Yan's seven-
volume treatise *Yi Xue Ru Men* (Introduction to Medicine),
published in 1575 A.D., distinguishes between *lao* and *zhai*, as
lao is heat in nature and belongs to the disease of *yang*, and
zhai is deficient in nature and is a disease of *yin*. *Yi Xue Ru
Men* also specifies six key symptoms: tidal perspiration, cough,

spermatorrhea, bloody urine, turbid urine, and diarrhea. According to *Yi Xue Ru Men*, if the symptoms appear in alternation, the conditon is still a mild one. When they appear concurrently, the condition is grave.

Classical scholars are in general agreement as to the etiology and pathogenesis of *lao zhai*. As has been noted, it is considered to be the consequence of infection by external evils or by contact with another person who has been so infected. However, there are significant contributing factors: excess in any of the seven emotions. *Qi qing* (seven emotional responses, identified as joy, anger, anxiety, worry, grief, apprehension, and fright), which can disrupt the normal functioning of all five organs, particularly spleen and kidney, and excess in sexual activity, which can debilitate *jin* (sperm) and *xue* (blood).

The clinical manifestations of *lao zhai* also conform to patterns of *yin* and *yang*. *Yin* deficiency symptoms are *gu zheng lao re*, low-grade fever, night sweating, sensation of heat in palms and soles, *sheng huo* ("flushing up"), cough, fatigue, and progressive emaciation. *Yang* deficiency symptoms are spontaneous sweating, sensation of chill, drowsiness, speaking in a consistently low voice, and fine, weak pulse. Most *lao zhai* sufferers manifest deficiencies in both *yin* and *yang*.

It is evident that the classical definition of *xu lao* and *lao zhai* syndromes apply to a number of ailments recognized by modern medicine: tuberculosis, severe hypoferric anemia, aplastic anemia, late-stage leukemia, leukopenia, and systemic lupus erythematosus, to name a few. AIDS conforms more closely and dramatically to the classical description than any other above-mentioned disease. Using the theoretical base and diagnostic approach of Traditional Chinese Medicine, it is possible to treat patients according to their *xu lao* or *lao zhai* symptom patterns, regardless of specific etiology or medical identification.

Principles and Therapeutic Measures

Beacuse *xu lao* diseases (including *lao zhai*) always affect several organs, differential diagnosis must be employed to determine which organ has suffered the most serious damage, whether deficiencies in *qi* (vital energy), *xue* (blood), *yin*, or *yang* are present, and whether *pi* (spleen) or *shen* (kidney) is the more deeply impaired. Only with this information in hand can an appropriate treatment plan be formulated.

The basic principles involved in treating *xu lao* and *lao zhai* are threefold:

Deficiencies must be remedied with tonifying herbal formulas.

Asthenia must be relieved by invigorating the body with warming herbal formulas.

Shen (kidney), the congenital source of *qi* (vital energy), and *pi* (spleen), the postnatal source of *qi*, must be nourished.

According to these principles, specific formulas were devised for each *xu lao* condition. (The ingredients for these formulas can be found in Appendix 3).

* *Xin Lao* (Heart Asthenia)
  da-wu-bu-wan (Major Five Organs Tonifying Formula)
  tian-wang-bu-xin-dan (Ginseng and *Zizyphus* Formula)
  suan-chao-ren-tang (*Zizyphus* Combination)

* *Gan Lao* (Liver Asthenia)
  fu-gan-tang (Liver-Tonifying Combination)

* *Fei Lao* (Lung Asthenia)
  bai-he-gu-jin-tang (Lily Combination)
  ren-shen-huang-ji-san (Ginseng and Astragalus Formula)

* *Shen Lao* (Kidney Asthenia)
  jia-wei-liu-wei-ti-huang-wan (Modified Rehmannia
  Six Formula)
  da-bu-yuan-jian (Major *Yuan Qi* Tonifying Formula)
* *Pi Lao* (Spleen Asthenia)
  xiang-sha-liu-jun-zi-tang (*Saussurea* and Cardamon
  Combination)
  shen-yang-yi-wei-tang (*Yang*-Lifting and Stomach-
  Nourishing Combination)
  zhi-sheng-jian-pi-wan (Ginseng and Dioscorea Formula)
* *Yin* Deficiency
  cheng-yin-li-lao-tang (*Yin*-Lifting and *Lao*-Nourishing
  Combination)
  da-bu-yuan-jian (Major *Yuan Qi* Tonifying Formula)
* *Yang* Deficiency
  cheng-yang-li-lao-tang (*Yang*-Lifting and *Lao*-Nourishing
  Combination)
  shen-fu-tang (Ginseng and Aconite Combination)

In addition, special treatments were devised for the *lao zhai*
condition. Emphasis was placed on measures to improve the
patient's emotional and psychological condition, to be taken
before any more specific program was adopted. Actually, these
measures were no more than common-sense advice: to regulate diet and health habits, to abstain from sexual activity, to
avoid emotional excess (particularly in giving way to anger or
fear), and to maintain a positive attitude toward one's own
ability to overcome the disease. But particular formulas were
recommended for certain symptom patterns characteristic of
lao zhai.

* Asthenic fever and night sweating (to be treated according
  to the principle of nourishing *yin* and clearing heat)
  qin-jiao-bie-jia-san (*Chin-chiu* and Tortoise Shell
  Formula)
  huang-qi-bie-jia-san (Astragalus and Tortoise Shell
  Formula)
  bie-jia-ti-huang-tang (Tortoise Shell and Rehmannia
  Combination)
  qing-gu-san (*Chin-chiu* and Rehmannia Formula)
  bao-zheng-tang (*Kao-ben* and Cnidium Combination)
* Asthenic dry cough, asthenic lung fire
  tai-ping-wan (Pacific Formula)
  nin-fei-tang (Lung-Tranquilizing Combination)
* Asthenic diarrhea
  shen-ling-bai-zhu-san (Ginseng and Atractylodes
  Formula)
  bai-zhu-gao (Atractylodes and Citrus Formula)
* Spontaneous and night sweating
  huang-qi-san (Astragalus Formula)
  shen-ji-san (Ginseng and Astragalus Formula)
* *Yang* deficiency, prolonged disease course
  bu-zhong-yi-qi-tang (Ginseng and Astragalus
  Combination)
  shi-quan da-pu-tang (Ginseng and *Tang-kuei* Ten
  Combination)
  ren-shen-yang-rong-tang (Ginseng Nutritive
  Combination)

To these formulas were frequently added ingredients
derived from animals: turtle shell (*Amyda sinensis, pieh-chia*),
turtle shell plastron (*Amyda sinensis, pieh-chun*), tortoise shell
(*Chinemys reevesii, kuei-pan*), gecko (*Gekko gecko, ge-jie*), deer

horn glue (*Cervus elaphus, lu-jiao-jiao*), and dried human placenta (*Homo sapiens, zi-he-che*).

Most of these classical formulas are still in use, modified in accordance with individual symptom complexes and contemporary research in the pharmacological effects of the constituents of herbs used in the formulas. The treatment principles and formulas we are using for AIDS treatment are based on the theories cited above and combined with the modern pathological and pharmacological research on AIDS and herbs. The modern pathophysiological research on *xu zheng* (*xu lao* and *lao zhai* belong to *xu zheng*) has further revealed that the nature of *xu zheng* is an imbalance of the immuno-endocrinological system.

Xu Zheng and the Disturbance of Neuroendocrine and Immune Functions

From its inception, the People's Republic of China has vigorously pursued the integration of Western and Traditional Chinese Medicine, with special emphasis on experimental research designed to test the scientific validity of traditional medical concepts. One of these, *xu zheng* (asthenic or deficiency conformation), encompassing *xu lao* and *lao zhai*, has been studied in connection with modern immunology, endocrinology and autonomic nervous-system theory (Liu et al. 1985; Jianhua Wang et al. 1986).

For more than 20 years, research in China has been directed toward translating the clinical manifestations upon which Traditional Chinese Medicine is based into scientific terminology through investigation of the objective pathophysiology involved. *Xu zheng* (asthenic or deficiency syndromes) has been a major focus of these studies. Most of the work has been done from the perspective of immunodeficiency and disturbances of the integration network within the hypothalamus for neuroendocrine and immune functions. As a result, it has been substantially demonstrated that the TCM diagnostic standard for *xu zheng* (see Appendix 1) is valid for the diagnosis and treatment of persons suffering from diseases whose symptoms, whatever their causes, fall within the range of *xu zheng*. This would seem to be particularly applicable to the HIV-ARC-AIDS phenomenon, whose pathophysiology remains unclear but whose manifestations correspond very well to the *xu lao/lao zhai* development described in the classical literature of Traditional Chinese Medicine. The remainder of this chapter will be devoted to the findings of research terms investigating kidney, spleen, lung, heat, vital energy, blood, and *yin* and *yang* deficiencies in terms of their neuroendocrine and immune functions, as recorded by modern testing procedures.

Kidney Deficiency

As diagnosed by the *xu zheng* diagnostic standard, elderly patients usually show kidney deficiency (KD) either in kidney *yang* (KDYa) or in kidney *yin* (KDYi). A recent survey of persons aged 60 or over at Shanghai Second Medical University found that 43.2% could be diagnosed as KD. Laboratory test figures for their endocrine and immune functions were compared with those for persons not diagnosed as KD (Xiang Xia et al. 1987).

A study of the effect of tonifying kidney on the immune function in the elderly (65 years and older) patients was performed by Shen and Wang. They found that the function of suppressor T-cell, Concanavalin A- (Con A) induced lymphocyte transformation and PHA-induced lymphocyte transformation were lower in the elders than in the young. After kidney-tonifying treatment, the three parameters of the elderly were improved and approached to those of the younger cases (Ziyin Shen and Wang 1987). With the use of kidney and spleen tonics, the clinical signs of kidney and spleen deficiencies disappeared. Laboratory tests showed an increase in NK cell and lymphocyte transformation and a decrease in plasma immunocomplex in both kidney and spleen tonifications, which suggested that the two regimens could activate the immune function.

Endocrinological studies of hypothalamus-pituitary-thyroid and gonad axis functions of KD patients, especially those diagnosed KDYa, found occult functional disorders in varying degrees at various levels in these endocrine axes. According to TCM theory, these disorders could be ameliorated by warming kidney *yang*. (Some young KDYa patients underwent changes identical to those observed in older patients, suggesting that KDYa produces the effect of premature senility.) KDYa patients were found to have lower thyroid function, and their T-3, T-4, and thyroid-stimulating hormone (TSH) levels were lower than those of non-KDYa persons (Gang Shi et al. 1986). In addition, both KDYa and KDYi patients were found to have diminished cyclic adenosine monophosphate/cyclic guanosine monophosphate (cAMP/cGMP) ratios and lower phagocytosis activity (Jigen Huang et al. 1987). AIDS patients show obvious kidney deficiency and also a high incidence of premature senility. Its constitutional changes may, therefore, be the same as those of the elderly or those of young KDYa patients.

The basic ingredients of kidney-tonifying formulas are epimedium, *Cuscuta*, and mahonia leaf for patients with KD of both *yin* and *yang*. For formulas for KDYa only, add aconite; for KDYi only, rehmannia is added.

Changes in KD patients match the dysfunction of the integration network in the hypothalamus which is responsible for neuroendocrine and immune functions. It follows that kidney-tonifying formulas can be expected to have a favorable effect on the functioning of this network (Gaoshang Fu et al. 1983).

Spleen Deficiency (SD)

Similar results have been reported for cell-mediated immunity in spleen *qi* deficiency (SQD) patients. One study found that the percentage of T-cells in circulating lymphocytes was 32.85±7.48%, significantly lower than normal. In regard to humoral immunity, immunoglobulins IgG and IgM were found to be 11.73±5.238 g/l and 1.284±0.543 g/l respectively, again well below normal limits (Zhenghua Li et al. 1987). Zhang reported that about 30-40% of SQD patients have a reduced number of or evidenced reduced activity in their circulating T-cells (Yuexuan Zhang et al. 1983; editorial of *Chinese Journal of Integrated Traditional and Western Medicine*, 1985).

A study of electrophoresis changes in lymphocytes of SD patients found that the electrophoretic rate in a group of 33 such patients was 0.777 ± 0.094, much lower than the normal 0.975±0.082 ($p < 0.01$). Slow electrophoretic rates were measured at 0.669±0.045, as compared to normal 0.714±0.0 3 ($p < 0.01$). It was concluded that the normal human lymphocyte is a kind of heterogeneous cell group with varying electrophoretic abilities, and that spleen deficiency is characterized by changes in that heterogeneity, resulting in lower lymphocytic electrophoretic ability and disorder in the distribution of fast and slow electrophoretic lymphocytes. This may be one of the mechanisms of reduced immunological function in cases of spleen deficiency (Yuanliang Kuang et al. 1988).

Spleen deficiency patients also show impairment in their digestive functions and immunity, as well as disturbances of their autonomic nerve functions. Substantial changes in the important regulating factors of cyclic adenosine monophosphate (cAMP), cyclic guanosine monophosphate (cGMP), and thymine deoxyriboside, as isolated by hydrogen radioisotope (H^3-TdR), were recorded in studies of 24 SD patients (Yin et al. 1985; see Table 2-1). These figures showed that SD patients have substantial changes in these important regulating factors.

Table 2-1 Comparison of SD Patients and Normal Persons

	Normal Control	SD Patients	P
cAMP	22.58±5.72 (n=39)	10.01±3.21 (n=24)	<0.001
cGMP	6.15±1.68 (n=42)	5.72±2.83 (n=24)	>0.05
cAMP/cGMP	3.67	2.54±1.76	<0.01
3H-TdR LCT	38038±18296	7092±6887.26	<0.001

Table 2-2 Comparison Before and After Treatment for Eight Cases with SD (*Qi* Stagnancy Reduced to *Qi* Deficiency)

	Before	After	P
cAMP	11.58±3.05	23.83±7.33	<0.001
cGMP	4.82±1.68	6.13±5.43	>0.05
cAMP/cGMP	2.83±1.69	5.85±3.23	<0.05
3H-TdR LCT	11458.25±9747.13	34515.6±24664.05	<0.05

After treatment with combined modern and Traditional Chinese Medicine, 14 of those cases were followed up; in 8 of these, the original *qi* stagnancy in the diagnostic standard symptom pattern was reduced to *qi* deficiency, and in the remaining 6, the entire spleen deficiency had disappeared (see Tables 2-2 and 2-3).

Table 2-3 Comparison Before and After Treatment for Six Cases in Which SD Symptoms Disappeared

	Before	After	P
cAMP	11.48±3.01	26.16±6.82	<0.01
cGMP	4.02±1.03	9.22±3.16	<0.05
cAMP/cGMP	4.30±3.22	3.09±1.08	>0.05
3H-TdR LCT	17550.10±7293.94	26285.67±7112.82	<0.05

The leading factor in SD conformation appears to be the cAMP, which regulates the differentiaton of cells and the tranformation of lymphocytes. When the cAMP level is low, cell differentiation and lymphocyte tranformation are suppressed, impairing immunity and possibly increasing the risk of cancer (Yin et al. 1985; Zhenghua Li et al. 1987; Jinsuan Jing et al. 1987).

Lung Deficiency (LD)

In TCM theory, lung *qi* is one of the chief sources of *zheng qi*, which is very important in resisting exterior evils. Although two other diagnostic standards have been divised for the identification of lung deficiency (one by the National Conference on Chronic Bronchitis, held at Guanzhou in 1979, the other by Yuling Qi and his colleagues in 1983), the standard followed here will be that of the National Committee for Integrating Chinese and Western Medicine in China (see Appendix 1).

The pathophysiological changes associated with LD have been determined to be as follows:

* Decrease of immunity, both in cell-medicated and humoral sections
* Low levels of cAMP and α_1-AT in the blood

* Vagotonia
* Reduced ventilation
* Increased resistance of passages
* Reduced blood flow in the lungs
* Rheological changes in the blood
  (He 1985).

Decrease in immunity has been demonstrated by the markedly lower number of T-cells and B-cells and percentage of T-cells in circulation patients diagnosed LD as compared to the normal population. Similarly, studies in Guangxi province showed a lower level of humoral immunity as determined by rate of lymphocyte transformation, globuline in the blood, IgM, and IgG in LD patients. These findings are all consistent with TCM theory, which adds that persons found to have LD are particularly vulnerable to invasion by exterior evils. Like AIDS, ARC, and HIV(+) patients, they are susceptible to frequent attacks of the common cold, influenza and sinusitis.

LD also lowers such functional regulating factors as cAMP, cGMP, and the ratio between them, and such energy metabolism factors as red blood cell content of ATP. This indicates that LD is a syndrome involving multiple organs.

The kidney, spleen, and lung are the most important organs in immunodeficiency syndromes, and most symptoms of persons with AIDS, ARC, and HIV infection coincide with the symptom patters of these three organs.

Yin and Yang Deficiencies (YiD, YaD)

A double-blind study of 87 typical YiD and YaD patients of Shanghai Traditional Medical College measured the body temperature, pulse rate, and blood pressure of patients who had previously been differentiated according to the xu zheng diagnostic standard. Average figures for *yang* deficiency patients were much lower than those for *yin* deficiency patients (p<0.001). As YiD and YaD symptoms were relieved by TCM treatment, a parallel reduction in the difference between these measurements was observed. When the results of previous studies of saliva pH levels and galvanic skin response (GSR) were taken into consideration, the findings matched Wenger's differentiation of sympathetic and parasympathetic nervous reaction types. It was concluded that the differentiation of YiD and YaD is closely related to the functioning of the autonomic nervous system (Yang and Kao 1987).

Immunologically, patients with YiD and YaD symptoms manifest reduced lymphocyte transformation under the stimulation of phytohemagglutinin, signifying a possible decrease in cellular immunity. Both groups show lower cell-mediated immunity than that found in normal persons with YaD patients registering even lower than YiD patients.

Endocrine functions in YaD patients have also been studied. To determine the functioning of hypothalamus-pituitary-adrenal (HPA) axes in these patients, the adrenal hormone glucocorticoid(GC) and its glucocorticoid receptor (GCR) in target cells were used as criteria. Both GCR in white blood cells and HPA axes were found to be significantly lower than normal in cases of *yang* deficiency (Jiaqing Zhang et al. 1987). In a parallel animal study, dopomine-beta-hypdroxylase (DBH) activity of the adrenal glands and brains in rats with experimentally-induced *xu han* (asthenic cold) and *xu re* (asthenic heat) was measured. *Xu han* was found to correspond with a decrease in DBH activity, *xu re* with an increase (Yuehua Lian et al. 1987).

Yin and *yang* are two opposite conditions in TCM theory; *yin* deficiency and *yang* deficiency are the clinical expressions of their respective weaknesses. In 9 cases of hyperthyroidism and 17 cases of hypothyroidism, it was found that their clinically-defined syndromes corresponded to the diagnostic standards for *yin* deficiency and *yang* deficiency, respectively. Analysis of their cAMP/cGMP ratios showed a predominance of cAMP in YiD and of cGMP in YaD (Ankuan Kuang et al. 1979; see Table 2-4).

Table 2-4 cAMP and cGMP in YiD and YaD Patients

	cAMP(pmol/ml)	cGMP(pmol/ml)	Ratios
YiD	16.0±1.3	7.4±0.73	71.0±1.25
YaD	29.9±4.1	4.7±0.66	2.60±0.32
Control	23.9±5.3	6.6±7.20	4.95±0.04

Further study of cAMP/cGMP ratios in *yin* and *yang* deficiencies in other Western-defined diseases in the *qi yin* deficiency syndrome and in the *yin yang* deficiency syndrome has generally borne out similar results (Zongqin Xia et al. 1979).

Although *yin* deficiency and *yang* deficiency are conceptual terms, their clinical manifestations are concrete, and the body of research that has been reviewed here has furnished a means of monitoring their treatment with considerable scientific accuracy. Experimental research has supplied more and more measurable figures to describe them. The treatment for these conditions will have a more accurate monitoring criteria.

Yin, yang, qi, and blood deficiencies are major symptom patterns in AIDS, ARC, and HIV (+) patients. But these deficiencies, as well as deficiencies of *qi,* blood, and all five organs, are also confirmable by clinical trials of herbal treatments. For example, when a *qi* tonic, which has been used for years to cure *qi* deficiency, is given as a treatment in a modern clinic with successful results, it may be inferred that the condition of *qi* deficiency was present in the patient who received it. And although *yin* and *yang* deficiencies in *qi* and blood (QD, BD) are so frequently associated that they may be suspected in most such cases, *qi* deficiency is usually found with *yang* deficiency, while deficiency in blood is usually found with *yin* deficiency. (The latter also manifests the symptoms of anemia.)

The laboratory findings reported earlier showed a definite tendency that the observable figures in the immune, endocrine, and autonomic nervous systems revealed the nature of *xu zheng* patients. Studies of the several symptom patterns of *xu zheng* (kidney, spleen, lung, *qi*, blood, *yang*, and *yin*) began by objectifying the symptom pattern, then determining the pathophysiological changes common to patients having the same *zheng* diagnosis but different diseases (in the modern sense), and confiriming the *zheng* parameters by comparing these patients with others whose diseases were the same but whose *zheng* diagnoses were different. Finally, prescriptions corresponding to the *zheng* were administered and the results observed.

The purpose of these studies was to determine which Chinese herbs possess the effect of regulating body homeostasis. For example, the regimen for tonifying kidney can regulate hormonal levels, the affinity of the receptor, and cellular and humoral immunity, while simultaneously enhancing the target hormone level without suppressing hypothalamus or pituitary function.

These studies clearly show that traditional Chinese Medicine, when used in tandem with modern Western research, can provide a solid foundation for treating civilization's most recent affront to good health – AIDS.

3

TCM Symptomatology and Conformations of AIDS, ARC, and HIV Infection

Introduction

The corpus of Traditional Chinese Medicine has been accumulated and substantiated through observation, experiments, and clinical trials. It is not based on empirical knowledge alone, but is a system developed in the distant past by individual scholars and government institutions. Many of the principles and remedies first advanced centuries ago have now been confirmed by modern science.

Since there were no laboratory tests in ancient times, clinical observation was the only available means for making diagnoses and evaluating the efficacy of treatments. Collecting and analyzing data concerning symptoms is the most important process in Chinese medical practice. Thus, Chinese medicine can be seen primarily as a medicine of symptomatology, the details of which will be discussed in this chapter, with special attention given to the symptoms of AIDS and their meaning in Chinese medical diagnosis and treatment. Clinical monitoring and prognosis will be discussed in a later section.

Eight principles are used to summarize clinical symptoms: *yin* or *yang*, exterior or interior, hot or cold, and deficiency or excess. In addition to these principles, there are analytical rules: three etiologies (external, internal, and neither external nor internal factors), differential diagnosis by analysis of the state of five solid organs, and analysis and differentiation of the diseases according to the state of vital energy (*qi*) and blood. The result of the diagnostic differentiation is a summary of the pattern of symptoms, called the *zheng* (symptom complex) or conformation in Chinese medicine.

A *zheng* is not the equivalent of a single symptom or even a series of symptoms. It is a TCM diagnostic unit. Although it begins with the analysis of symptoms, the cause, the position, the nature of the illness, and the response of the patient to the treatment are all taken into account in reaching a diagnosis. The diagnosis of a conformation, therefore, reveals the essence of the total state of disorder rather than the diagnosis of a specific disease (Shen 1987).

From the conformational point of view, AIDS can be classified as an extreme form of deficiency in spleen, lung, and kidney. Depending on its progression, it can cover a whole spectrum of *xu lao* (deficient) conformations, from slight fatigue to exhaustive consumption or "wasting away" – the *lao zhai* discussed in the previous chapter.

Since AIDS is a syndrome, not a distinctive disease, the clinical manifestation of AIDS includes many symptoms of its complications. The subjective symptoms and objective signs vary with the complications and their severity. Although AIDS patients have certain common symptoms, none of them is specific to AIDS. Roughly, we can divide these symptoms into two major categories: constitutional symptoms and symptoms of various complications.

Constitutionally, there are certain symptoms which represent the whole body condition, or the overall reaction of the body to pathogenic agents. They are not specific to any particular pathogen or disease, but are indicative of the patient's general health. A pale complexion, pale tongue, weak pulse, low energy level, shortness of breath, fatigue, body and muscle aching, low grade tidal fever, a sensation of chill, cold limbs, a sensation of heat in palms and soles, spontaneous or night sweating, emaciation, poor appetite, and emotional instability are all symptoms that can occur in a number of different diseases. The point of TCM constitutional diagnosis and therapy, however, is to treat the whole person rather than to treat his or her disease. It is true "health care" rather than "disease management" (Dharmananda 1986); it evaluates the patient's constitution in diagnosing a condition and has developed systematic treatments for the various constitutional changes which may occur. Although constitutional therapies of this kind stand in opposition to much of modern medical practice aimed at the treatment of diseases, and thus will be perceived as a type of "complementary practice," since the founding of the People's Republic of China, Chinese physicians have been combining the constitutional and allopathical approach with considerable success.

Symptoms characteristic of AIDS are so-called opportunistic infections and specific types of malignant tumors which are usually not found in people with normally functioning immune systems. These ordinarily innocuous or rare complications come in five categories: cancers, parasitic infections, viral infections, fungal infections, and bacterial infections (Douglas et al. 1987). They are manifestations of the collapse of the body's immune functions and are usually the first indication that the patient has probably contracted HIV. The most common infection is *Pneumocystis carinii* pneumonia (PCP) and the most common cancer (or cancer-like condition) is Kaposi's sarcoma (KS). Together these account for most of the fatalities attributed to AIDS in the United States. Symptoms of these opportunistic diseases are specific, and they are sometimes decisive evidence for an AIDS diagnosis. However, in the asymptomatic initial stage of HIV infection, clinical observation is relatively useless, and the only way to determine whether a person is infected is to perform a blood test.

The Integration of Western (Disease) and TCM (Conformation) Diagnostic Approaches

Traditional Chinese Medicine identifies sickness by deducing the overall functioning of the human body from a macroview of the entire system. It diagnoses a sickness by analyzing the patterns of the symptoms, or the symptom complex, the *zheng* (conformation). Western medicine, on the other hand, has based its development on the foundation of modern science, using experimental research and microscopic evidence to identify a sickness from a microview of a specific part or parts of the body. Chinese and Western medicine see the same disorder from different viewpoints, each having its own features, significance, and advantages.

Integrating the Western diagnosis of disease and the TCM diagnosis of conformation to formulate a better a scheme of treatment is a popular and effective practice in China's health care system. Using both kinds of diagnostic information and treatment has yielded much more efficacious therapeutic results than has been achieved by either in isolation.

To exemplify this approach, we can look at AIDS. Western medicine has found its causative virus and the mechanisms of the viral infestation – the destruction of the

T-4 cells by the AIDS virus, thereby incapacitating the body's immune functions. This information is essential in formulating the treatment strategy, since we know that treatment must not only be antiviral, but must also rebuild the human immune system. Thus the Chinese medical practitioner can search for the correct herbs, those which have antiviral and immuno-enhancing effectiveness, but if there were no medical evidence from Western medicine, Chinese medicine would not have these clues to take into account in formulating the correct treatments. Contemporary pharmacological research on the antiviral and immuno-enhancing or regulating effects of various herbs have also made available information which is essential in selecting and formulating effective herbal combinations. Such pharmacological data will be discussed more fully in Chapter 7.

On the other hand, to date, Western medicine has provided no cure for AIDS, since in Western medicine, a cure means the total elimination of the pathogen and the damage it has caused. Current treatments offered by Western medicine, such as AZT, only serve to slow the disease progress or alleviate some of the symptoms. Since Western medicine is aimed narrowly at the virus, it delegates little effort to means which might aid the body's recuperation or, more broadly, foster the patient's general health.

Alternately, in TCM, health is defined as the maintenance of the body's balance, both internally and with its external environment. Fitness is the goal of TCM treatment, which emphasizes the normalization of the body's functions and has developed a systematic way to treat patients according to their own conformations. Integrating the two medical philosophies enables one to benefit from both approaches while minimizing the shortcomings of either one.

Investigation of the patient's conformation is based on clinical standards established by TCM theory. For the diagnosis of *xu zheng* (asthenia), the Sub-Committee on Deficiency and Aging of the National Committee for Integrating Chinese and Western Medicine of the People's Republic of China has set up a standard for the *xu zheng* (deficient conformations). The first version of this standard, established at the Guangzhou conference in 1982 (Shen 1987), was revised at the Zhengzhou conference in May 1986. Since AIDS, ARC, and HIV (+) patients can definitely be assigned to various deficiency conformations. This revised standard is found in Appendix 1.

In order to integrate the two kinds of diagnostic information, we must understand the specific methods used in TCM diagnostics, namely the so-called "four examinations": inspection, auscultation and olfaction, inquiry, and palpation (in common terminology, seeing, hearing and smelling, questioning, and touching). Only by combining the four can the disorder be systematically comprehended and a correct diagnosis be made.

Inspection

Inspection is the observation of the patient's expression, color, appearance and tongue.

● Expression

Expression is the outward manifestation of the vital activities. Expression of spirit in TCM means whether *shen* (spirit) exists. Loss of *shen* means lack of vigor and is a serious omen of a poor prognosis. Generally speaking, if the patient is in fairly good spirits, behaves normally with a sparkle in the eyes and keen response, and cooperates with the doctor during the examination, the disorder is mild. In our clinical experience with AIDS/ARC and HIV (+) patients, most asymptomatic HIV (+) patients manifested such an expression. Although when first diagnosed as positive, they tended to feel anxious and to be in low spirits, this period usually passed, and they were then able to calmly face the facts and begin coping. Most of them even felt more aware of meaning in their lives than they had previously and became more alert in order to combat their infection.

If the patient is spiritless, indifferent in expression, with dull eyes and a sluggish response or even experiences mental disturbances and so does not cooperate during the examination, the disease is serious. Most AIDS/ARC patients in the advanced stages are in such a situation, especially those with infections located at the central nervous system or those who have collapsed from extreme fatigue. When facing impending death, the typical AIDS patient shows exuded vital spirit and a total loss of *shen*.

- Color

People of different races have different skin colors, and there is wide variation among people of the same race; however, a lustrous skin of its characteristic color is considered normal. A normal complexion is slightly dark, but lustrous and ruddy. Morbid complexions vary: red, which denotes the existence of heat; pallor, which indicates the existence of cold or deficiency of blood; bright yellow, which suggests jaundice; and bluish purple, which is often due to stagnation of blood or severe pain.

Most AIDS/ARC patients tend to have a wan, pale, sallow, and emaciated complexion. When the disorder advances to a critical stage, the face looks like dried bone; pallor and lack of luster – the color of extreme deficiency of *qi* and blood – is apparent. When the patient has a PCP infection, a dark-gray color, as if the face were covered with dust, overshadows the pallor. In most hepatic complications, the face looks as if it were covered with dirt; even if jaundice is present, the yellow is not bright, but grayish yellow – *yin* yellow in TCM terminology. The faces of patients with KS and other lymphoma often manifest a blue, purplish color. Patients with miliary tuberculosis and other chronic respiratory system infections sometimes show focused red spots on their cheeks, especially in the afternoon, when they feel a "flushing up." The fingers and toenails of AIDS/ARC patients sometimes become gray- or black-striped. This is a sign of blood deficiency and stagnation.

The color of such excretions, as nasal discharge, sputum, stool, urine, and vaginal discharge, is also symptomatic. Clear or white excretions generally denote deficiency and cold, while those that are turbid and yellow indicate heat or excess. Discharges of AIDS/ARC patients usually belong to the former condition; only intermittently, when they have episodes of infection, do these excretions temporarily become excess in color.

● Appearance

The patient's bodily condition, posture, and movement need also be observed. The obvious symptoms in AIDS/ARC patients are wasting away and muscular atrophy, like that usually seen in chronic consumptive diseases. At the very late stage, there is evidence of profound constitutional disorder, marked by general ill health and malnutrition, a state of cachexia. Patients with brain infections, such as encephalitis and meningitis, have severe problems with motor coordination. TCM describes this condition as pathogenic wind and sputum conformation.

● Tongue

Observation of the tongue, including both the tongue proper and its coating, is an important procedure in TCM diagnosis. A normal tongue is of an appropriate size, light red in color, free in motion and with a thin layer of white coating over the surface, which is neither dry nor overly moist. In AIDS/ARC and HIV(+) patients, the predominant tongue signs are pale or purple pigmentation, puffiness, and obvious tooth marks on the margin (scalloped tongue). When the disorder has advanced to a critical stage, the tongue coating becomes blackish and dry and the tongue tissue's color becomes dark red with an enlarged congested sublingual vein. In patients with *Candida*, the tongue coating becomes white, thick, and sticky, and can be removed by a Q-tip. In patients with hairy leukoplakia, the lesions (usually at the sides of the tongue) are the over-growing filiform papillae, and cannot be removed. When patients have emotional disturbances, or there is asthenic heat, the tip of the tongue becomes red.

Auscultation and Olfaction

It is important to listen to modes of speech, respiration, and coughing. In general, uttering sounds that are feeble or in an extremely low tone indicates a deficiency conformation. Feeble breathing accompanied by shortness of breath and sweating after slight exertion usually indicates *qi* deficiency. In AIDS/ARC patients, these are common symptoms.

Smelling a discharge or excretion can also differentiate excess and deficiency, in AIDS/ARC patients, since the odor of most of their discharges is insipid. Their phlegm is usually flat in odor and white in color, which indicates the deficiency.

Questioning

Questioning is asking the patient or the patient's companion about the disease condition in order to understand its pathological process. Questions to be asked include both the patient's own chief complaints and the traditional *shi wen* (ten questions).

● Chief Complaints

Since AIDS is a syndrome, different patients and/or the same patient at different stages register various chief complaints. The complaints are one of the important factors to consider in formulating the appropriate herbal combinations. The most common chief complaints are fatigue, low-grade fever, mouth infections, skin lesions, shortness of breath, diarrhea, body aching, mood swings and frequent respiratory tract infections. The onset, duration, and past history of each complaint are also important to note.

Questioning also means asking about ten conventional symptoms. The first is chills and fever. In AIDS patients, there are two kinds of chills: those preceding a high fever, as in an episode of pneumonia, and those resulting from an extremely low energy level. The first kind of chill is a indication of invasion by wind-cold (an infection); the second condition indicates *yang* deficiency. In both cases, a reduction in the intensity or duration of the chill can be an indication that the energy level is rising.

There are three kinds of fever in AIDS patients. A high fever, such as the fever accompanying an acute episode of PCP, is one in which the temperature is 102° F or higher. From the viewpoint of TCM, this results from the invasion of wind-cold or wind-heat. The second kind of fever, the one most commonly encountered in AIDS patients, is a low-grade tidal fever, in which the temperature reaches around 101° F in a recurring, tide-like pattern. This kind of fever occurs in patients who have persistent flu-like symptoms and is associated with tuberculosis, or *Mycobacterium avium-intracellulara* (MAI), a condition attributed, in TCM theory, to endogenous heat, to *yin* deficiency, or to a residual fever which has not been cleared by the initial treatment. The third type of fever, usually seen in the late stages of AIDS and in patients with disseminated TB or MAI infections, is a "false" fever with no increase in body temperature. It is characterized by a sensation of heat rising to the face ("flushing up"), a sensation of heat in the palms and soles, and/or *gu zheng lao re* (literally, "debilitating heat steaming from the bone"). In TCM theory, this is a sign of severe *yin* deficiency.

Inquiring about perspiration is also important in diagnosing AIDS patients. Their mildly abnormal perspiration pattern is characterized by frequent spontaneous sweating exacerbated by slight exertion, which is a sign of *yang* deficiency. AIDS patients also frequently complain about profuse sweating during the night, which is an indication of *yin* deficiency. In the terminal stage of AIDS, profuse cold sweating is a sign of exhaustion of both *yang* and *yin*.

Inquiring about appetite and taste yields information about gastro-intestinal functioning, or in TCM terminology, the condition of spleen *qi*. A good appetite, meaning that the body system is digesting food well and that there is a desire to eat, shows the postnatal source of *qi* (vital energy) is still efficacious. When patients lose their appetites, spleen *qi* is deficient, and the treatment should first concentrate on rebuilding spleen *qi*. TCM theory holds that when the body is too deficient, tonification can not be effective. Since tonification is a major component in the treatment of a disease like AIDS, improving spleen *qi* is usually the initial step of TCM treatment of AIDS. If a patient complains of stickiness or a sweet taste in his or her mouth, it is a sign that there is retention of food and water in the stomach, resulting in dampness in the spleen.

Bowel movement in AIDS patients is also an important symptom to be noticed. AIDS patients rarely complain of constipation unless they are extremely deficient in body fluids and essence. Diarrhea, however, is a common complaint. Loose stool and chronic diarrhea are signs of spleen deficiency; diarrhea in the early morning with the passage of undigested food is a sign of deficiencies in both spleen and kidney. Occasionally, acute gastritis, incurred by eating contaminated food, will produce diarrhea together with pain and a sensation of heat. TCM considers this to be a condition of dampness-heat in the intestines. Parasitic infections, such as amebiasis and cryptosporidiosis can cause persistent severe diarrhea, the symptoms of which yield a TCM diagnosis of combined spleen and kidney deficiency and dampness-heat blended to the lower energizer.

The color and quantity of urine is used as an indication of whether the patient's conformation is cold or hot. A yellow color is a sign of heat; clear and profuse urine is a sign of cold and deficiency. Most AIDS patients have clear and profuse urine. Frequent nocturia is a sign of kidney deficiency.

Pain is another of the ten questions. Persistent flu-like body and muscle aches are common complaints of AIDS patients. If it can be relieved by pressure or by warmth, the pain is deficient and cold in nature. The location of the pain is an indication of which inner organ is involved. Pain above the diaphragm indicates the disorder of heart and lung; pain in the epigastric region indicates disorders of spleen and stomach;

pain in the lumbar region, around and below the umbilicus, means kidney disorders; pain in the costal and hypochondriacal region indicates disorders in liver.

The patient's patterns of sleep and emotional states should also be investigated. Insomnia accompanied by dizziness and palpitations usually indicates failure of the blood to nourish the heart because of deficiency in both heart and spleen. Insomnia accompanied by mental restlessness and dream-disturbed sleep indicates hyperactivity of heart fire. AIDS patients with neurological symptoms usually show memory loss and disorientation; in TCM theory this is attributed to an accumulation of phlegm-dampness.

Female patients must be asked about their menses and any other vaginal discharges. The frequency and duration of the menstrual cycle and the quantity, color, and odor of the discharge are all helpful in determining whether the patient's conformation is one of excess or deficiency.

Palpation

Although palpation may be exercised on other parts of the body as well, the term most frequently is applied to feeling the pulse at the wrist. The radial artery throbs will be felt by three fingers, divided into three corresponding regions: *cun*, *guan*, and *chi* (see Fig. 3-1). The region opposite the styloid process of the radius is known as *guan*, that distal to *guan* (i.e. between *guan* and the wrist joint) is *cun* and that proximal to *guan* is *chi*. The three regions of *cun*, *guan*, and *chi* of the left hand reflect, respectively, the conditions of heart, liver, and kidney, and those of the right hand reflect conditions of lung, spleen, and kidney.

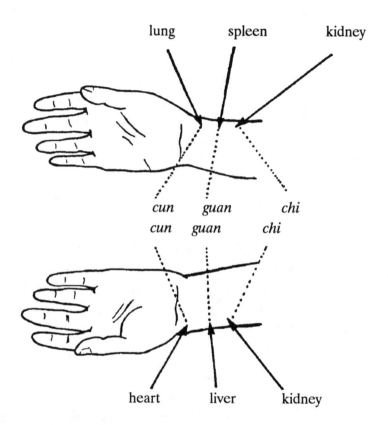

Fig. 3-1 The Three Regions For Feeling Pulse

A normal pulse is of medium frequency (four to five beats per breath) and regular rhythm. It is even and forceful.

A superficial or floating pulse can be felt when pressed lightly, becoming weak or completely absent on heavy pressure. This often occurs in the early stages of HIV infections, when the patient has obvious flu-like symptoms. It can also occur in a chronic prolonged course of HIV infections, which indicates a general weakness or deficiency.

A deep or submerged pulse can be felt only by heavy pressure. It often occurs in AIDS patients, because AIDS is primarily a interior conformation.

A slow pulse with fewer than four beats per breath often accompanies a general sensation of chill and a very low energy level.

A rapid or fast pulse can usually be felt in cases of infectious complications (tuberculosis, MAI, viral cardiomyositis).

For a *xu* (deficient) type person, the pulse is weak and forceless and disappears upon heavy pressure. This is the most common type of pulse in AIDS, ARC, and HIV (+) patients. Especially when it is fine and thready, it indicates *qi* and blood deficiency conformations of AIDS patients. A thready pulse at the *chi* position indicates kidney deficiency.

The foregoing are the most common pulse types in AIDS patients. When two or more types of pulse are felt in one patient, it is important to make a comprehensive analysis of the clinical significance of these combinations, while taking into consideration the general condition of the patient.

In order to collect the symptoms systematically, to keep a good record, and to enable the integration the of symptoms into conformations, we designed a chart to be used in our clinical trial (see Table 3-1).

This chart not only provides TCM diagnostic information, but also some conventional medical information. Since we work with patients who have been already diagnosed and treated by conventional medicine, this conventional information is necessary to know and to follow up when we communicate with their physicians and monitor the progress of their treatment.

Table 3-1 Chart for Recording Symptoms
Clinical Record Form (Initial Visit)

RECORD# _____ Date: (M/D/Y)_____

Patient's Name: _____ Sex: (M/F) _____

Date of Birth: (M/D/Y) _____ Occupation: _____

Marital Status:

Married _____ Divorced _____ Single _____

Sexuality:

Gay _____ Heterosexual _____ Bisexual _____

IV Drug Use:_____ Blood Products Contact: _____

Mailing Address: _____

Telephone: Day: _____ Evening: _____

WORKING

Full-time _____Hours Per Week _____ Not Working _____

AIDS _____ARC _____HIV(+) Date diagnosed(M/D/Y) _____

Protozoal infections: PCP(M/D/Y) _____

    Toxoplasma gondii encephalitis (M/D/Y)_____

    Cryptosporidium enteritis (M/D/Y) _____

    Isospora belli (M/D/Y) _____

Viral infections: Herpes simplex (M/D/Y) _____

    Herpes zoster (M/D/Y)_____

    Herpes genitalis (M/D/Y)_____

    Cytomegalovirus (CMV)(M/D/Y) _____

    Multifocal leukoencephalopathy (MLP)(M/D/Y)_____

    Hepatitis B (M/D/Y)_____

    EBV (M/D/Y) _____

Fungal infections: candidiasis (M/D/Y)_____

Cryptococcal infection (M/D/Y) _____

Bacterial infection: TB (M/D/Y) _____

MAI (M/D/Y) _____

Cancers: Kaposi's sarcoma (KS) (M/D/Y) _____

Non-Hodgkin's lymphoma (M/D/Y) _____

STD: Syphilis (M/D/Y) _____

Gonorrhea (M/D/Y) _____

Others: Hairy Leukoplakia (M/D/Y) _____

Lymphadenopathy (M/D/Y)_____

MAIN SYMPTOMS

Fever _____Night Sweats _____ Chills _____

Fatigue_____Weight Loss _____ Malaise _____

Diarrhea_____Poor Appetite_____ Shortness of Breath ____

Insomnia _____Memory Loss _____ Muscle Pain_____

MAJOR PHYSICAL SIGNS

T_____P_____R _____BP_____

Height:_____Weight: _____ Skin lesions:_____

TCM SYMPTOMS

Expression

Good Spirits _____Spiritless_____Disturbance _____

Complexion

Normal_____Pale _____ Lustrous_____

Lusterless_____Red_____ Yellow _____

Bluish purple_____

Physical Appearance

Emaciated _____ Normal _____ Obese _____

Tongue

Normal_____ Pale _____ Deep Red _____

Purplish _____ Flabby _____ Thorny _____

Deviated_____ Cracked _____ Scalloped _____

Sub-Lingual Vein Congestion _____

Tongue Coating

White _____ Thin _____ Thick _____

Wet_____ Dry_____ Yellow _____

Thin _____ Thick _____ Wet _____

Dry_____ Grayish Black _____ Thin _____

Thick _____ Wet _____ Dry_____

Peeled _____ Mirror _____ Geographic _____

Voice

Low Volume ___Normal _____ High Volume_____

Inquiring

Fever   Fever _____ Chills _____

Cough   Cough _____ Shortness of Breath ____

Sweating   Spontaneous Sweating _____

                  Night Sweating _____ Profuse Cold Sweating __

Thirst   Thirsty _____ Prefers Hot Drinks_____

                  Cold Drinks_____ No Desire to Drink_____

                  Not Thirsty _____

Appetite	Poor Appetite_____	Foul Belching _____
	Retention of Food _____	Sweet Taste _____
	Bitter Taste_____	
Bowels	Constipation _____	Loose Stools _____
	Diarrhea _____	With Undigested Food__
	Early Morning Diarrhea _____	
Urine	Deep Yellow_____	Clear and Profuse _____
	Frequency _____	Nocturia_____
Pain	Persistent_____	Headaches_____
	Lingering_____	Chest _____
	Upper Abdominal _____	Lumbago _____
	Lower Abdominal_____	General Body Aching___
Mental	Insomnia _____	Drowsiness _____
	Memory Loss _____	Disorientation _____
Menstrual	Short Cycle _____	Prolonged Cycle _____
	Deep Red _____	Light _____
	Excessive_____	Scanty _____
	Leukorrhea _____	Yellow Thick_____
	Pre-menstrual Syndrome _____	
	White Thin _____	
Pulse		
	Lung _____	Spleen _____
	Heart _____	Liver_____
	Kidney_____	Floating _____
	Deep _____	Slow _____
	Rapid_____	Wiry_____
	Thready_____	Weak _____
	Strong _____	

Others

Ringing in Ears_____Dizziness _____

Low Sex Drive _____

TCM DIAGNOSIS

Qi Deficiency _____Blood Deficiency_____

Yin Deficiency_____*Yang* Deficiency_____

Lung Deficiency _____Spleen Deficiency _____

Kidney Deficiency ____Heart Deficiency_____

Liver *Qi* Depression_____ Asthenic Heat _____

Heat Steaming From Bone ____ *Qi* Stagnancy ____

Blood Stagnancy_____*Shen* Disturbance _____

Accumulation of Dampness and Phlegm _____

Dampness Heat _____Other:_____

LAB TESTS

P24_____ Beta-2 Microglobulin _____

T-Total: _____ T-4 ____T-8 _____ T-4/T-8 _____

CBC: WBC_____% Lymphocyte_____

RBC_____HCT _____

CONVENTIONAL MEDICATIONS

AZT _____DDI _____

Alpha Interferon_____

Pentamidine Isethionate_____

Bactrim _____Septra_____

Other_____

REFERRING M.D. or D.O. _____

HISTORY: Diseases_____

Allergy _____

Family_____

MEDICAL INSURANCE _____

Evaluation of Symptoms and Conformations

The objective evidence and indications of clinical status obtained by TCM's four diagnoses are further analyzed and synthesized into an appropriate diagnosis. In Traditional Chinese Medicine, each of these symptoms is related to the conformations which have been described and for which treatments have been developed for thousands of years, and these treatments have been enhanced by recent pathophysiological and pharmacological research findings.

● Deficiency Conformations

Most HIV (+) and ARC patients show the symptoms and signs of deficiency, particularly as deficient conformations of kidney, spleen and lung. In AIDS the symptoms are not fundamentally different, but include more deficient heat, blood stagnation, and *shen* disturbances (Misha Cohen 1986). Although not every AIDS or ARC patient has all these symptoms, the symptoms of patients with certain kinds of complications are usually fairly consistent. Therefore, TCM conformations for AIDS and ARC patients can be clinically considered as sub-types of the disorder. Generally, deficiency conformations can be catalogued as *qi*, blood, *yin*, and *yang* deficiencies. Any of these deficiencies can combine with another deficiency in a particular organ to become a combined deficiency conformation. In AIDS patients, the most commonly affected organs are lung, spleen, and kidney.

● Spleen Deficiency

If the patient's symptoms are predominantly located in his or her digestive system, with diarrhea, loose stool, stomach distention, poor appetite, weight loss, lack of energy, and a complexion with a yellow tinge, the patient has spleen deficiency.

Since spleen deficiency usually co-exists with *qi*, *yin* and *yang* deficiencies, we need to investigate whether the patient has any of these conditions as well.

● Spleen *Qi* Deficiency

If in addition to the foregoing symptoms, the patient has low spirits, fatigue, shortness of breath, low voice, spontaneous perspiration, a corpulent or "scalloped" tongue, and weak and powerless pulse, the patient has spleen *qi* deficiency. All the symptoms of *qi* deficiency commonly exist among ARC and AIDS patients. This is a stage of dysfunction of the gastrointestinal system.

● Spleen *Yang* Deficiency

If in addition to symptoms of spleen deficiency, the patient is reluctant to speak and has chills either in his or her whole body or in certain parts of the body, edema in face or feet, pale and corpulent tongue with moist coating, sinking, slow and indistinct pulse, and a large amount of colorless urine, the patient has spleen *yang* deficiency. Spleen *yang* deficiency is the further development of spleen *qi* deficiency. It implies that dysfunction of the gastrointestinal system has become more severe.

● Spleen *Yin* Deficiency

If in addition to the symptoms of spleen deficiency, the patient has dry lips and throat and thirst without appetite for food, constipation or dry stools, red tongue with little coating or without coating, fine and fast pulse, "flushing up" in the afternoon, and ulcers in the mouth and on the tongue, the patient has spleen *yin* deficiency. This is a deficiency of body fluids (blood, *ye*, and *jing*), which implies an even more advanced stage of spleen deficiency. At this stage, the patient shows a great deal of deficiency heat.

The most severe spleen deficiency combines spleen *yin* and *yang*. All of these stages have been observed in our clinical experiences with ARC and AIDS.

* Diarrhea

In AIDS patients, diarrhea, the dominant symptom of spleen deficiency, has several sub-types, the most common of which may be noted here.

Diarrhea caused by deficient spleen *qi* can be identified by a watery stool, undigested food in the stool, and other symptoms of deficient spleen *qi*.

Diarrhea caused by deficient kidney *yang* and spleen *qi* is distinguished by an early-morning need to defecate, sparse, watery stool, cold limbs, and other symptoms of kidney deficiency.

Diarrhea caused by stagnant food is a frequent form of diarrhea in AIDS patients, because it involves the functioning of the lower GI system. The symptoms are sticky and foul-smelling stool, and distention of the epigastrium and abdomen.

● Lung Deficiency

If the majority of the patient's symptoms are found in the respiratory system, with shortness of breath, susceptibility to the common cold, and prolonged coughing episodes, the patient has lung deficiency. Most AIDS and ARC patients with respiratory system complications in the chronic stage manifest these symptoms. (The acute phase of respiratory infections in the early stage of the AIDS has a different pathogenesis and should be treated differently. It will be discussed later.)

Since lung deficiency usually co-exists with *yin* and *qi* deficiencies, these deficiencies should be explored.

● Lung *Qi* Deficiency

If in addition to the symptoms of lung deficiency, spontaneous perspiration, a pale complexion and tongue, and a weak pulse are noted, the patient has lung *qi* deficiency.

● Lung *Yin* Deficiency

If in addition to the symptoms of lung deficiency, a dry cough, dry throat, bloody sputum, temporary loss of voice, red cheeks, "flushing up", emaciated appearance, and a sensation of heat in the palms and soles are present, the patient has lung *yin* deficiency. This condition is usually seen in patients in the advanced stages of AIDS and ARC, especially when complications like tuberculosis and MAI have arisen.

● Acute Lung Infections

When AIDS or ARC patients are invaded by respiratory infections such as PCP in the early stage of the disorder, their physical constitution is still relatively strong and the symptoms are likely to be quite different. At first, dramatic reactions to the *Pneumocystis carinii* infection include high fever, chest tightness, nonproductive cough and shortness of breath, indicating an excess lung heat conformation. This stage can be treated by antibiotics, such as cotrimoxazole, but the patient will continue to be subjected to frequent relapses because of the underlying immunosuppression. The TCM therapeutic principle for this stage is to clear lung heat and nourish the lung *yin* using the methods discussed in the following chapter.

● Kidney Deficiency

Either because of their former lifestyles (sexually active or IV drug using), or simply because of the nature of AIDS virus infection, most AIDS and ARC patients have very obvious kidney deficiency symptoms. Even in HIV (+) persons, a weak *chi* pulse is a very common sign. Their sexual drive is also diminished, sometimes to the point of impotence. Most patients experience lassitude in the loins and legs, numbness in the legs, lower back pain, ringing in the ears, hair loss, floccose gums, and a frequent need to urinate during the night. Kidney deficiency is a very common conformation among AIDS and ARC patients.

● Kidney *Qi* and *Yang* Deficiency

If in addition to the foregoing symptoms, chills in the whole body, especially from the waist down are noted, the patient is suffering from deficiency of kidney *qi* and *yang*. Other symptoms are a blackish complexion, a subdued, quiet manner, low spirits, sterility, spermatorrhea, hearing loss, copious, clear urine, and edema. The tongue is corpulent, "scalloped", and pale with a thin, moist, white coating. The pulse is generally weak and submerged, especially at the *chi* position.

Many AIDS or ARC patients in a relatively chronic stage of the disorder experience these symptoms. They usually feel cold and want to be in a warm place; if they are thirsty, they would rather have a hot drink than a cold one. This means that their general energy level is low. In TCM, kidney *qi* and *yang* are the sources of congenital vital energy and their deficiencies deplete all bodily functions.

● Kidney *Yin* Deficiency

If in addition to the symptoms of kidney deficiency, patients have a thin, shriveled constitution, persistent thirst, a dry mouth, a sensation of heat in palms, soles, and chest (in TCM terms, *wu xin fan re,* literally, heat in the five centers), reddish cheeks, "flushing up" in the afternoons, night sweating, hearing loss, impotence, memory loss, and dizziness, kidney *yin* deficiency can be diagnosed. The tongues of these patients are red or dark red with little or no coating. The pulse is thready and fast. When AIDS and ARC reach their advanced stages, these symptoms are frequently present.

Deficient *yin* causes deviation in the inner balance: the body manifests symptoms of heat, "flushing up", a sensation of heat in five centers, and thirst. Heat of this kind is not a real heat; patients usually complain that they feel hot inside their bodies at the same time that feel cold on the surface. This is an internal deficiency-heat syndrome, a hectic fever due to *yin* deficiency, and is a common conformation in advanced stages of AIDS and ARC.

● Combined Multi-Organ Deficiencies

Especially at the advanced stages of AIDS and ARC, many patients have gastrointestinal, respiratory, and nervous system complications, as well as lymphadenopathy and other malignancies. Combinations which are likely to occur are spleen and lung *qi* deficiency, spleen *qi* and kidney *yang* deficiency, lung *qi* and kidney *yang* deficiency, lung and kidney *yin* deficiency, and *qi* and blood deficiencies in the lung, spleen, and kidney simultaneously. The terminal stage of AIDS is characterized by extreme deficiency (collapse, or wasting away) of *qi* and blood in all organs.

Conformations Other than Deficiencies

● Stagnant *Qi* and Blood

The primary symptom of stagnant *qi* and blood is distention in the chest or abdomen, often with palpable lumps, pain, and soreness. Tumors, lumps, hard masses, and skin lesions are also very common in AIDS/ARC patients. The patient's complexion tends to be of a dark purple tinge; the tongue is dark purple, sometimes with red spots, and the sublingual vein is congested. The pulse is usually choppy. Such symptoms are very common in patients with KS and lymphadenopathy. Although, according to TCM theory, these are conformations of excess, when they occur in AIDS/ARC patients they become false sthenia conformation in appearance but true asthenia conformation in nature.

● Hindrance of *Chinglo* by Phlegm-Dampness Stagnation

Lymphadenopathy, lymph node swelling, and lymphosarcoma are common malignancies in AIDS/ARC patients. In TCM, these nodules are attributed to the dysfunction of the spleen and the accumulation of phlegm and dampness. Central nervous system symptoms caused by toxoplasmosis or encephalitis also contribute to the accumulation of phlegm. In TCM this is called confusing the heart openings (*tan-mi-xin-qiao*), the impairment of consciousness caused by invasion of phlegm to the heart, which causes the pathologic changes of unconsciousness and mental confusion, disorientation, coughing with rales, coma, chest distress, whitish, glossy coating of the tongue, and slippery pulse.

The TCM diagnosis of the patients we treated in the San Francisco AIDS Alternative Healing Project can be used as a group of examples, although the number is not large enough to represent a general distribution of the conformations of AIDS, ARC, and HIV (+) patients. Divided according to their diagnosis of HIV infection, their TCM conformations are shown in the following three histograms.

HIV (+) patients appear to have more *qi*-, blood-, and liver-related conformations, suggesting greater emotional instability.

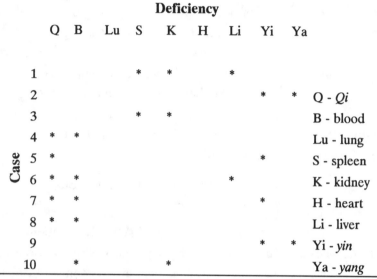

Deficiency

	Q	B	Lu	S	K	H	Li	Yi	Ya
1				*	*		*		
2								*	*
3				*	*				
4	*	*							
5	*					*			
6	*	*					*		
7	*	*						*	
8	*	*							
9								*	*
10		*			*				

Case (rows 1–10)

Q - *Qi*
B - blood
Lu - lung
S - spleen
K - kidney
H - heart
Li - liver
Yi - *yin*
Ya - *yang*

Fig. 3-2 Multi-Organ Deficiencies in Ten AIDS Patients*

*AIDS patients all had multi-organ deficiencies, with *qi*, blood, and *yin* deficiencies being the most common.

The number of patients represented in Figures. 3-3 and 3-4 are too small to be more than suggestive of a generalized pattern.

Deficiency

	Q	B	Lu	S	K	H	Li	Yi	Ya
1				*	*				
2	*	*							
3					*				
4	*								
5				*					
6				*			*		

Case (rows 1–6)

Fig. 3-3 Deficiencies in Six ARC patients

* ARC patients had less multi-organ involvement and less *yin* deficiency.

Deficiency

	Q	B	Lu	S	K	H	Li	Yi	Ya
1								*	
2							*		
3	*	*						*	
4								*	
5	*	*							
6	*	*				*			

(row labels at left: "Case" spanning rows, values 1–6)

Fig. 3-4 Deficiencies in Six HIV (+) Patients

Ascertaining the distribution of the conformations of AIDS, ARC, and HIV (+) patients can help us to develop better formulas. For such a widespread epidemic, TCM treatment measures must have a certain generalizability of application, but also a certain specificity in order to meet the immediate clinical needs of the individual patient. In a patient-care clinical setting, individualization is the key to better therapeutic results; this is possible only through an accurate diagnosis of each patient's conformation.

4

TCM Clinical Therapeutics for HIV Infections

Integrating TCM and Western Treatments

In our discussion of AIDS diagnosis in the previous chapter, it was mentioned that integration of the Western diagnosis of a disease with the TCM diagnosis of a conformation will give us a better understanding of the disease and of the patient's general health. For the treatment scheme, we also should combine these two approaches, formulating herbal therapies according to TCM differential diagnosis of the patient's *zheng* without neglecting the pathogenic factors to be discovered by Western medical techniques. In this way, we can utilize the pharmacological value of herbs in both traditional and modern understandings.

Allopathically, Western drugs are very specifically directed at attempting to eradicate the AIDS virus, and the opportunistic infections and cancer cells associated with the virus. At this time, however, these drugs have not been successful at accomplishing these goals without the high cost to the patient of toxic side effects which prevent long-term use or seriously limit their dosage. If we can use TCM herbs to compensate for these side effects, the therapeutic effects of Western drugs can be enhanced. TCM herbal treatment and other comprehensive measures are focused upon the constitutional condition of the patient, and so are relatively nonspecific; however, they can definitely improve the patient's general condition so that the body is better able to combat pathogens.

Western medical research has provided some understanding of the pathogenic changes resulting from HIV infection. On the basis of that understanding, the treatment of AIDS/ARC or HIV (+) patients can benefit from a number of TCM strategies. One is the use of antiviral herbs to reduce the potency of the virus. Another is the use of herbal immune regulators to rebuild the immune system. Thirdly, herbs can be used more specifically to treat the whole spectrum of opportunistic infections and malignancies related to AIDS/ARC. These measures may improve the quality of life for the years the patient has left or even prolong the patient's life span by reducing the incidence or intensity of life-threatening complications. Curtailment of the multitude of potentially life-threatening opportunistic diseases reduces the "cofactor" effects which so frequently accelerate the progress of the HIV infection. Finally, herbs can be used to compensate for the side effects of Western medications, such as the anemia caused by AZT. Their supportive effects can both enhance the therapeutic potency of such medication and mitigate those side effects.

AIDS and other chronic viral infections sometimes have much more far-reaching influences on the patient's constitutions. Viruses (unlike bacteria, for which effective therapies exist) always appropriate the biosynthetic apparatus of the host cell, so that, for example, drugs effective against viruses tend to damage mammalian cells (Gallo 1988).

TCM's basic principle is always to treat the patient's entire constitution, and immunodeficiency is decidedly a constitutional pathogenic change. Good results have been reported in the treatment of immunodeficiency other than AIDS, resulting from organ transplants, cancer therapies, and viral infections (Dong 1978; Hanbing Huang 1982; Jiang 1979; Lin Li 1983; Liao 1982; Jinglan Liu 1983; Lou 1983). These experiences can be used as guides for the treatment of AIDS.

Western medicine has produced few immune-enhancing drugs. TCM, however, has a long history of dealing with deficiency conformations which are clearly related to immunodeficiencies (see Chapter 2). The relationship of TCM deficient conformations and immunodeficiency has been proved by many scientific studies. TCM strongly emphasizes the adjustment of bodily functions, including the enhancement of the body's natural ability to defend itself against pathogenic invasion (*zheng qi*). Tonification is a chief treatment measure of TCM and most tonics have immuno-enhancing and regulating effects (see Chapter 7).

There are Western drugs which can be used for the treatment of opportunistic infections, but AIDS/ARC patients need to be able to use them on a long-term basis, perhaps the duration of their lives. Because their natural immunity has been damaged, the relapse rate after discontinuing these drugs is almost 100%. Opportunistic infective fungi, protozoa, and bacteria exist everywhere and can be contracted easily; therefore, new infections will take place continuously. The drugs used to treat these infections should be of extremely low toxicity and without obvious side effects. TCM herbal treatment has proven very effective and the herbs are virtually without serious side effects (Hsu 1989).

A controversy exists about the treatment of cancerous complications due to an AIDS infection. Most Western anti-cancer drugs have immune-suppressive effects, which are definitely undesirable for use by a patient with an already badly damaged immune system. From long-term experience in treating cancer with TCM, practitioners in the People's Republic of China have found that integrating Western and TCM treatments brings the most successful therapeutic results (Yan Sun et al. 1987).

TCM Herbal Formulas

In centuries of clinical experience, TCM doctors have learned to compound herbal formulas on the basis of the properties and flavors of individual herbs in order to deal with diseases of different natures. Chinese herbal formulas are usually composed of between eight and twelve different herbs. The combination of these component herbs is called an herbal formula, and the science of the composition, action, indications, dosage, and clinical uses of these herbal formulas is called herbal pharmaceutics.

A Chinese herbal formula is generally composed of four classes of herbs: imperial, ministerial, assistant, and servant. The imperial herb is the chief herb of a formula; the ministerial herb is ancillary to the imperial herb; the assistant herb augments the actions of the preceding two herbs or diminishes their side effects; the servant herb coordinates and directs the actions of all the herbs comprising the formula. From long-term clinical practice, some standard formulas, called basic formulas, have emerged. The addition or omission of herbs to or from these basic formulas results in different effects.

In this book we will introduce some basic formulas we designed and used in our experimental clinical trials at the San

Francisco AIDS Alternative Healing Project and in our later clinical trials at Integrated Health Services in Lakewood, California, and discuss their effects and applications. Basically there were three groups of formulas: formulas directed toward the root causes of AIDS, i.e. antiviral and immuno-enhancing formulas, formulas to relieve constitutional symptoms, and formulas directed toward specific complications of AIDS.

The most common criticism of herbal medicine is that herbs are not stable in respect to their active essence, since species, collecting seasons, and production sites are likely to vary. Furthermore, the method of preparation (drying, steaming, decocting) may dilute the active essence of the herb (Hsu 1988). Finally, it is objected that herbal medicine is inconvenient to prepare for ingestion. However, variables can be reconciled through scientific preparation procedures to achieve a consistent pharmacological effect, and extracts can be concentrated to the point that the daily dosage is small and requires no special preparation. Before prescribing any formula, the practitioner should first determine whether its manufacturer exerts an acceptable level of control over the nature and quality of the raw materials and the procedures followed in their processing.

The treatment of HIV infection should follow the TCM treatment principle for chronic deficiency conformation (*xu lao*). Because complicated mechanisms are involved in the pathogenesis of these deficiency conformations, the treatment should first differentiate between the principal and the secondary aspects of the illness and the acute and the chronic episodes of the complications.

In AIDS, the deficiency is usually secondary to the HIV infection, so that the HIV infection is the principal and the asthenia a secondary manifestation. If the patient is not very asthenic (deficient), the treatment should concentrate on the HIV infection, with the antiviral (*quxie*) principle as the main mode of attack. If asthenia is the major manifestation, the treatment should first focus on tonifying the deficiency. Of course, both aspects of the disorder may be treated at the same time.

When an AIDS patient has a new episode of infectious complications, the asthenia becomes the principal and the new acute infection the secondary aspect. In this case, the treatment should first focus on the acute new infectious condition and only afterwards take care of the chronic asthenic condition.

The above-mentioned principle of treatment is a very important TCM clinical rule and is termed "treating the *biao* (secondary) aspect for emergency and the *ben* (principal) aspect for chronicity."

When more than one organ is involved in a conformation, for instance, if spleen and kidney are both involved, the asthenia of spleen and kidney should be seen as the principal and the other organs' asthenia as the secondary aspects. Which organ should be treated first depends on which aspect is in the acute phase. Therefore, herbal treatment for AIDS should differentiate between the acute and chronic, the principal and the secondary aspects of the conformation in order to formulate an appropriate scheme of treatment. Only in this way can we ensure progress from deficiency to a normalized condition.

As we have indicated in the previous chapters, AIDS, ARC, and HIV (+) patients belong to the category of deficiency conformations. The general principle of treatment for a deficiency is tonification. In applying tonification to specific cases, the status of *qi*, blood, *yin*, *yang*, and the organs involved must be taken into account. This method is especially useful in treating the constitutional symptoms of HIV-infected persons. For simple deficiencies, such as simple *qi*, blood, *yin*, or *yang* deficiency, the treatment is to invigorate the *qi*, blood, *yin*, or *yang*. For deficiencies involving multiple organs, the relationship between these organs should also be taken into consideration.

There are three kinds of tonification formulas. Potent tonifiers are suitable for rapid-developing deficiencies; mild tonifiers are suitable for chronic, long-lasting deficiencies; and balanced tonifiers are suitable for mild deficiencies. In treating HIV infections, HIV (+) patients are most likely to benefit from balanced tonifiers; in the relatively stable stage of AIDS/ARC, mild tonifiers are most effective. Only when the deficiency becomes very severe should potent tonifiers be used.

Tonification is an important measure for treating the constitutional conditions of AIDS patients. But we also take into consideration the scientific and medical evidence in selecting herbs, i.e. we try to select herbs on the basis of their pharmacological natures and the pathogenesis of the disorder (Yong Zhou et al. 1985). In addition to tonifying herbs, therefore, anti-pathogen and anti-cancer herbs are considered in devising formulas for an AIDS patient.

In addition to episodes of opportunistic infections, malignant cancers are also known to develop. Intermittently, excess conformations are seen in AIDS patients, even though AIDS remains primarily a deficiency condition. These intermittent, false excess conditions must be perceived as asthenic conformations in both appearance and reality. When we try to use antiviral, anti-inflammatory, heat-clearing, and phlegm-expelling herbs, which are cold and purgative in nature, we must balance these formulas to prevent the patient who is actually asthenic from being harmed.

Since HIV (+) patients are, for the most part, asymptomatic, basic herbal treatments must be directed toward reducing the potency of the virus and enhancing the immune system as preventive measures against repetitive infections which can accelerate the progress of the infection. As these are basic antiviral and immune-enhancing treatments, they are also appropriate for ARC and AIDS patients.

Basic Treatments for HIV Infections

HIV Infection

AIDS, ARC and HIV(+) are three different stages of the HIV infection. Clinically, they tend to overlap each other. (The definitions of these conditions can be found in Appendix 2.) The HIV(+) stage means only that the patient has been infected by HIV and that HIV antibodies are present in his or her blood; there are no or very few clinical symptoms.

From a TCM conformational view, the three stages affect the *qi*, blood, *yin*, or *yang* of the five solid and six hollow organs. TCM diagnosis does not sharply differentiate between these three stages, concerning itself primarily with clinical manifestations of their symptoms.

Asymptomatic HIV Carriers

The CDC estimates that 1.5 million Americans have been infected by the HIV. The onset of the infection varies from person to person; most patients do not know exactly when the infection was contracted. The first signs of the infection are very similar to those of influenza or the common cold, but some patients do not manifest even these signs. From the TCM point of view, the typical onset is similar to the warm-

toxic disorder, a seasonal infectious disease described by the
Febrile Diseases School of TCM (Yu et al. 1987).

After the initial infectious reaction, most patients will
remain in an incubation period for anywhere from two to
twelve years. During this period, patients are generally in good
health and asymptomatic. Unless they are tested for HIV antibodies, it is difficult to distinguish them from HIV (-) people.
Eight HIV(+) patients, all male homosexuals, in our clinical
trial were in this category. When the project began in March
1988, it had been an average of 11.9 months (range: 3 to 21
months) since their first positive HIV test. All of them were
still working or studying full time, though their laboratory tests
showed substantial pathogenic changes, and one patient had a
positive P24 test. Their T-cell total count average was 854.3
(range: 352 to 1116; the normal average being 1600), their T-4
cell count average was 344.7 (range: 118 to 641; the normal
average is 944), and their T-4/T-8 ratio average was 0.63
(range: 0.3 to 1.56; the normal average range is 1.1-2.8).

TCM diagnostic observation revealed *qi* deficiency in
various degrees in most of these eight patients. When the
project started, six of them had puffy and tender tongue tissue
with obvious teeth marks ("scallops") on the margins of the
tongue. Some tongues were pale in color; a few tongues were
marked with purple spots, signaling blood deficiency or stasis.
Pulse palpation showed a very weak *chi* pulse (the pulse of
kidney) at both hands in four patients, and two of the patients'
chi pulses were very difficult to feel. Five of them complained
of chronic fatigue, three suffered from diarrhea, and two had
lost weight. Most of them reported a very low sex drive. Many
of these symptoms may be explained by previous lifestyles: excessive sexual activity surely would injure the body and impair
of the body's vital energy, especially kidney *qi*.

The principle of treatment for these patients is antiviral and immuno-enhancing. "Antiviral" in TCM terminology is *quxie* (eliminating external evils), and immuno-enhancing is *fuzheng* (supporting the body's natural order). If any constitutional symptoms are present, specific treatments for these special symptoms should be added.

From the TCM point of view, viral infections are the equivalent of invasion by the external evils of toxic heat and dampness. Antiviral or *quxie* treatment is designed to clear the heat and cool the blood, eliminating dampness and detoxifying the body. The selection of antiviral herbs is dependent on the relevant pharmacological data (see Chapter 7), the pathophysiology of the disease as defined by Western medicine, and the traditional use of heat-clearing and detoxifying herbs. Since most of these herbs are cold or purgative in nature, they should be well balanced by warm and tonifying herbs when they are used to treat HIV infections.

During our clinical trials, we developed a series of herbal formulas for treating HIV infection and its complications. These formulas have serial code names beginning with HY-. Among them, HY-30 and HY-31 were the most frequently used as the basic treatment. Their ingredients are as follows.

HY-30 *fuzheng & quxie* * - II

> viola, lonicera, epimedium, licorice,
> astragalus, ligustrum, ganoderma

HY-31 *fuzheng & quxie* - III

> viola, epimedium, coptis, prunella,
> licorice, astragalus, cassia seed

---

* *fuzheng*: supporting the body's natural order, i.e. enhancing immunity
* *quxie*: eliminating external evils, i.e. reducing the potency of the virus

HY-30 is a basic formula for all HIV-infected patients. Among the seven herbs in HY-30, viola, lonicera, epimedium, and licorice have exhibited inhibitory effects on HIV (Chang 1988; Barton 1989). In traditional TCM use, viola, lonicera, and licorice are main ingredients of a very famous traditional formula, Three Flower Combination (viola, lonicera, chrysanthemum, and licorice), used for the treatment of viral diseases such as mumps (Dinshan Chen 1942, 1987). Both on the basis of modern pharmacological research and in the light of traditional usage, these four herbs play a major antiviral role. The very bitter and cold property of viola and lonicera is balanced by epimedium and licorice. The other three herbs, astragalus, ligustrum, and ganoderma, are immuno-regulating herbs. The immuno-enhancing effects of these herbs have been demonstrated (see Chapter 7), as they are also traditional tonics for *qi*, *yin*, and kidney deficiencies. Epimedium is an important kidney *yang* tonic and also has immuno-enhancing effects.

The active component of licorice is glycyrrhizin (GL). Japanese researchers have found that GL appears to be effective in preventing an HIV infection from developing into the symptomatic stages. Long-term oral administration of GL to ten asymptomatic HIV-infected patients whose immunologic abnormalities, as described by Zolla-Pazner et al. (see Ikegami), ranged from 1 to 2 was effective in maintaining the infection in the asymptomatic stage. Neither progression of immunologic abnormalities nor development of HIV infection has been evidenced in a year's time. As regards the control group of patients not treated with GL, two patients developed AIDS (score 3) and died, while one has developed lymphadenopathy (score 3), but is alive, as of this writing (Ikegami 1989).

If the patient shows great emotional instability and liver disharmony, HY-31 is an alternative. The HIV-inhibitory herbs in this formula are viola, epimedium, coptis, prunella, and licorice. Coptis has inhibitory effects, not only on HIV, but also on a wide spectrum of bacteria and fungi. In TCM use, it clears away heart fire and tranquilizes the heart. Prunella also inhibits pathogenic germs and is especially successful against tuberculosis. Combined with cassia seed, it lowers ascending liver fire. When a patient seems to be emotionally unstable, this formula has a calming effect. The immuno-regulating herbs in this formula are astragalus, epimedium, and licorice.

HY-22 *fuzheng & quxie* - I

> astragalus, siler, ginseng, salvia,
> isatis leaf and root, rehmannia,
> deerhorn, *tang-kuei*, licorice,
> smilax, *Cuscuta*, millettia

HY-22 was designed and used in a previous SFAAHP clinical trial in 1988. Besides *fuzheng* and *quxie*, this formula also includes blood-activating herbs to promote the circulation of blood and expel stagnant blood. In this formula, the antiviral ingredients are isatis leaves and root. For specifically inhibiting HIV, they can be replaced by viola and lonicera. According to TCM theory, long-lasting diseases usually cause blood stasis. In our previous clinical trial, we found that most patients have stagnant blood, so when the patient shows the symptoms of blood stasis (dark red or purple tongue, congested sublingual vein), this formula should be used.

The following four formulas, designed and used in the previous SFAAHP trial, can also be used for antiviral and immune-enhancing treatment.

HY-1 *fuzheng* - I
bupleurum, scute, pinellia, ginseng, jujube, licorice, ginger, astragalus, siler

HY-2 *fuzheng* - II
astragalus, siler, ginseng, *Polygonatum* root, epimedium, rehmannia

HY-3 *quxie* - I
isatis leaf, bupleurum, *Lithospermum*, licorice, citrus rind

HY-4 *quxie* - II
isatis root, gardenia, blechnum, licorice, citrus rind

For *fuzheng* treatment, HY-1 and HY-2 can be used. If the patient has more symptoms of liver and spleen disharmony, HY-1 should be used. This formula is based on Minor Bupleurum Combination and the main ingredients of the Jade Screen Formula. The former is a harmonizing formula. Astragalus and siler are the main ingredients of the Jade Screen Formula, which has been studied in China as a major immuno-enhancer (Lu 1982). In traditional usage, siler usually accompanies astragalus to obtain a coordinating effect in strengthening defense *qi* (*wei qi*).

At the Fifth International AIDS Conference, Japanese researchers reported on Minor Bupleurum Combination's inhibitory effects on HIV reverse transcriptase. Their findings indicated that the activity of HIV reverse transcriptase was inhibited by more than 70% in the presence of 200 micrograms/ml of Minor Bupleurum Combination. The inhibition was dose-dependent, and the drug curtailed enzyme activity by 90% at 500 micrograms/ml, a clinically attainable concentration. Of the seven ingredients of Minor Bupleurum Combination, the extract from the radix of the plant *Scutellaria* was found to have a strong inhibitory effect on the reverse transcriptase activity at concentrations less than 50 micrograms/ml. In contrast to reverse transcriptase, cellular DNA polymerases α, β, and γ were much less sensitive to inhibition by this drug, supporting the contention that Minor Bupleurum Combination is non-toxic to the host cells (Ono 1989). Fujimaki et al. reported at the same conference that Minor Bupleurum Combination and Ginseng Combination improved the T-4/T-8 ratio and other immuno parameters in 7 of 13 patients treated (Fujimaki 1989).

HY-2 is designed to have tonifying effects on both *yin* and *yang*. Astragalus and ginseng are combined to tonify *qi* (*qi* belongs to *yang*); when combined with *Polygonatum*, they can especially strengthen spleen and lung *qi*. The *qi*-strengthening effect is enhanced by epimedium, which is a kidney *yang* tonic. Rehmannia and *Polygonatum*, when used together, are blood and *jing* (the main substances of *yin*) tonics. Epimedium and siler are inhibitors of various viruses and bacteria (see Chapter 7), and in general, all six of the substances contained in HY-2 have immuno-enhancing properties.

For *quxie* treatment, HY-3 and HY-4 can be used to reduce the potency of the virus. These two formulas can be used alternately to avoid any tolerance problems. For HIV infection, these formulas have less specificity than HY-30 and HY-31. They were designed before the HIV-inhibitory potency of certain herbs became public knowledge (see Chapter 7). In these two formulas, citrus rind and licorice are used to balance the cold and bitter properties of the antiviral herbs. When administered to HIV-infected asymptomatic patients, licorice has prevented or forestalled the development of AIDS (Ikegami 1989).

The prescribed administration of these formulas is as follows: the daily dosage is three grams three times a day, always on an empty stomach. When taking in powder form, three grams of the herbal powder are placed in the mouth and washed down with warm water. If capsules are used, six capsules containing 0.5 grams each are taken three times a day.

Single herbs can often be used to treat a disorder. In China, herbal injections are used in a variety of circumstances. For viral diseases in particular, injections of bupleurum, viola, and lonicera are common (Cao 1983). Hypericin, an alkaloid derived from hypericum, is now being tested for AIDS effectiveness in the San Francisco area (Hebert 1989). Hypericum has been extensively used for treating hepatitis B in China. (Detailed information about this herb can be found in Chapter 7.) Trichosanthin, the active constituent of *Trichosanthes*, has been tested and found effective in selectively killing HIV-infected lymphocytes and macrophages. (A detailed review of this herb will be presented by Qingcai Zhang in his upcoming book, *Trichosanthin: Its Clinical Applications*, to be published in mid-1990.) Another herbal product used in the treatment of AIDS is aloe vera, a Chinese herb whose healing ability has long been recognized. In Dallas, a clinical trial using the extract of aloe vera alone is reported to have enabled four-fifths of its subjects to return to work (reported in the July 12, 1988, edition of the *Dallas Times Herald*).

From the TCM point of view, however, a single herb is likely to cause side effects. For instance, aloe vera can produce unacceptable diarrhea. Formulas containing other herbs capable of balancing these effects are preferred.

Treatments for Constitutional Symptoms of HIV Infections

Constitutional treatments are used for treating systemic symptoms and improving the general health condition of AIDS/ARC or HIV (+) patients. As has been previously noted, HIV infection causes immunodeficiency in the body, and this deficiency is closely related to spleen, lung, and kidney deficiencies in Traditional Chinese Medicine. In a previous publication, Zhang reported on five groups of constitutional asthenic symptoms (Qingcai Zhang 1989). A more detailed discussion is appropriate here.

● Spleen Asthenia

Constitutional symptoms related to spleen asthenia (spleen deficiency) include poor appetite, loose stool, dyspepsia, a pale jaundice-tinged complexion, emaciation, weak pulse, and a puffy "scalloped" tongue. When these symptoms are present, the patient's chief complaint is usually gastrointestinal dysfunction.

The principle for treating spleen deficiency is tonifying *qi* and strengthening spleen, warming the middle energizer and dispelling cold, in order to invigorate gastrointestinal functioning.

Invigorating spleen and stomach is very important in the treatment of asthenic disorders. TCM holds that the spleen is the postnatal source of vital energy (*qi*), and only if spleen *qi* is functioning can the patient be treated for other symptoms. Strong gastrointestinal functioning is the prerequisite for the absorption of nutrition and the restoration of stamina. When the patient has a good appetite, the gastrointestinal system is functioning well, thereby promoting the desire to eat. If the patient has no appetite at all, the first step of treatment is to stimulate the appetite, thus enabling the patient to absorb the herbs prescribed for his condition. The following formulas can be used to treat spleen deficiency.

HY-10 *jian-pi** - I

> ginseng, atractylodes, hoelen, citrus rind,
> licorice, pinellia, *Saussurea*, cardamon

HY-20 *jian-pi*- II

> ginseng, ginger, licorice, aconite,
> atractylodes

HY-32 *jian-pi* - III

> ginseng, *Dolichos*, atractylodes, hoelen,
> dioscorea, lotus seed, coix, cardamon,
> platycodon, licorice

---

* *jian-pi*: invigorating spleen and stomach

HY-10 can be used when the dysfunction of the gastrointestinal function is mild, especially if poor appetite is the chief complaint. It is designed to treat weakness in the gastrointestinal system and to promote convalescence after a long-term illness. HY-10 is a modification of the Four Major Herb Combination, in which ginseng, atractylodes, hoelen, and licorice are the basic ingredients for strengthening the functioning of stomach and intestines. Citrus and ginseng increase appetite; pinellia, atractylodes, and hoelen dispel stagnant water in stomach and intestines; *Saussurea* eases abdominal pain and arrests diarrhea; cardamon relieves chest distention. Whenever poor appetite has become the major complaint, this formula should be used.

HY-32 can be used when gastrointestinal dysfunction has progressed to a more advanced stage, manifesting loss of appetite, diarrhea, fatigue, chills, abdominal distention, borborygmus, weak pulse, and anemia caused by long-term malnutrition. At this stage, the spleen *qi* deficiency has progressed and the patient shows few symptoms of spleen *yang* deficiency. This formula, also based on the Four Major Herb Combination, uses *Dolichos*, dioscorea, lotus seed, and coix to nourish spleen and stomach. Cardamon acts as a diuretic and improves stomach functioning. Platycodon nourishes stomach and treats diarrhea.

HY-20 can be used when the dysfunction of the gastrointestinal system becomes severe. In addition to the symptoms already mentioned, the typical symptoms of this stage are watery diarrhea with undigested food, early morning diarrhea, chills and fatigue, and especially a sensation of chill in the abdomen. The conformation for this stage is spleen and kidney *yang* deficiency. This formula is composed by adding aconite to Ginseng and Ginger Combination. Ginseng, ginger, licorice, and atractylodes nourish spleen *qi* and dispel chills. Aconite is a kidney *yang* tonic to warm the body by improving metabolic functioning.

Diarrhea is one of the common symptoms of spleen deficiency. If diarrhea lasts more than two weeks, a further clinical check is necessary to determine the cause. If it is a specific diarrhea caused by protozoa, CMV, or other pathogens, those formulas are not appropriate; diarrhea of this kind is a complication, not a constitutional symptom, and will be discussed in the following chapter.

The following are constitutional symptoms related to lung deficiency and asthenic lung heat: coughing, a sensation of heat in the chest, shortness of breath, fatigue, poor vocal production, reluctance to speak, red tongue, and a fast and fine pulse. An immune-compromised person is one whose respiratory system is constantly being re-infected by new pathogens. In TCM, this is a sign of defense *qi* (*wei qi*) weakness. Controlling chronic mild infections in the lungs and upper respiratory tract can reduce the burden upon the immune system and eliminate the cofactor effects of these inflammations.

The principle of treatment is clearing heat and nourishing lung. The following herbal formula should be used.

HY-7 *qing-fei-re** - 1

> scute, platycodon, morus, apricot seed,
> gardenia, asparagus, fritillaria, citrus rind,
> jujube, bamboo, hoelen, ginger, *tang-kuei*,
> ophiopogon, licorice, schizandra

---

* *qing-fei-re*: clearing heat from the lung

In HIV-infected persons, repeated infections of the upper respiratory tract is a prominent phenomenon of lung *qi* deficiency. Sinusitis, the common cold, and influenza persist longer in HIV (+) than in HIV (-) persons. Even after an initial treatment of the infection, the symptoms of a mild feverish sensation in the chest and unclear heat in the lung remain for a long time. This condition can be cleared up by HY-7. Platycodon and Fritillaria Combination, on which HY-7 is based, is designed to clear internal heat from the respiratory organs and treat symptoms like chronic inflammation, mild fever, cough, viscid phlegm, sore and itching throat, and hoarseness. In the formula, scute and gardenia remove internal heat in the chest. *Tang-kuei* and licorice nourish blood and subdue "flushing up." Asparagus, ophiopogon, and schizandra nourish lungs, remove internal heat from lungs, and relieve coughing. The remaining herbs coordinate and improve the effects of the other herbs.

If the fever is persistent and the temperature is higher than 101° F, an acute infection of the respiratory system is present. In this case, the patient should be advised to have a clinical check to see whether there is a specific infection. If so, the condition should be treated as a complication rather than a constitutional symptom. If no specific infection is found, this is a case of a false excess condition in an underlying deficiency disorder, and HY-8 or HY-33 (see following sections) should be used. These two formulas should be discontinued once the acute inflammation is cured or becomes chronic. In the latter case, these formulas should be replaced by HY-7.

● Kidney Deficiency

Kidney is the prenatal source of vital energy and the "root of life," since all other organic activities depend upon the kidney. As such, it is the most important organ in treating deficiency syndromes. In particular, sexual potency, bone marrow function, and water and *qi* regulation are all related to kidney. In patients with HIV infection, kidney deficiency has often been a predominant conformation.

Simple kidney deficiency or kidney *qi* deficiency is manifested in low sex drive, lassitude, sluggish gastrointestinal functioning, dysuria or polyuria, cold limbs, tinnitus, dark complexion, and a weak *chi* pulse. If this is the most obvious conformation of the patient, Rehmannia Eight Formula should be used. The ingredients of this formula are as follows.

Rehmannia Eight Formula

      rehmannia, cinnamon, aconite, hoelen,
      dioscorea, alisma, moutan, cornus

Kidney *yin* deficiency can be diagnosed by such symptoms as low-grade fever, night sweating, red cheeks, yellow urine, thirst, fast and fine pulse, and a red tongue with little coating. These symptoms show that there is asthenic heat caused by kidney *yin* deficiency. In this case, formula HY-16 should be used.

HY-16 *qing-xu-re** - I

> anemarrhena, phellodendron, hoelen, cornus, dioscorea, alisma, moutan, rehmannia

---

qing-xu-re: clearing asthenic heat

This formula is based on the Rehmannia Six Formula, a basic formula for nourishing kidney *yin*. Anemarrhena and phellodendron are added in order to purge fire and protect kidney *yin*.

● *Yin* Deficiency

Constitutional symptoms related to *yin* deficiency are chronic low-grade fever, anxiety, vexation, night sweating, and insomnia. If asthenic heat (low-grade fever) is the predominant symptom, the following two formulas can be used.

HY-18 *qing-xu-re*- II

> *chin-chiu, ching-huo*, mume, ginger, anemarrhena, *tang-kuei*, bupleurum, tortoise shell, lycium bark

---

HY-33 *qing-xu-re*-III

> gypsum, anemarrhena, oryza, licorice, ginseng

HY-18 is good for long-lasting low-grade fever caused by advanced lung and kidney *yin* deficiency. It is especially suitable for a type of fever described in TCM as *gu zheng lao re* (debilitating heat steaming from the bone). This formula is based on *Chin-chiu* and Tortoise Shell Formula, generally used for hyperplastic tuberculosis in which the major symptoms are low-grade fever, fatigue, flushed cheeks, night sweating, and progressive emaciation. *Chin-chiu* is antipyretic and can relieve the distressing symptoms of *yin* deficiency. Tortoise shell and anemarrhena nourish *yin* and rid the body of internal heat. Lycium bark and *ching-hao* remove the hidden fever and cool the blood. *Tang-kuei* is both a hematinic and a carminative. Bupleurum acts as an antipyretic and muscle relaxant. Mume is an astringent which inhibits sweating.

HY-33 should be used when the asthenic fever persists and the temperature is 101° or higher. Once the temperature is reduced to normal or lower, this formula should be replaced by HY-18. HY-33 is based on Ginseng and Gypsum Combination. Gypsum is a sedative and antipyretic, anemarrhena dispels internal heat, and ginseng is a tonic which compensates for the purgative effects of the first two herbs. Licorice and oryza are the harmonizers and are used as adjuvant herbs.

● Combined *Yin* and *Yang* Deficiencies

HY-34 is a formula traditionally used for night sweating caused by *yin* deficiency and asthenic fire. The action of the formula is to inhibit perspiration by nourishing *yin* and clearing heat. In these aspects, recent research has proved its effectiveness (Lianqing Shi 1982). *Tang-kuei* and rehmannia (both raw and prepared) nourish *yin* and blood, increasing the amount of body fluids and clearing heat. Coptis, scute, and phellodendron clear heat and relieve anxiety. Astragalus astringes the skin and inhibits perspiration.

Constitutional symptoms related to both *yin* and *yang* deficiencies are spontaneous sweating and night sweating. If *yang* deficiency is the more obvious manifestation and spontaneous perspiration is the chief complaint, HY-35 should be used. If *yin* deficiency is the more obvious symptom, with night sweating as the chief complaint, HY-34 should be used.

HY-34 *zhi-dao-han** - I

> *tang-kuei*, rehmannia, astragalus, coptis, scute, phellodendron

---

HY-35 *zhi-dao-han* - II

> astragalus, white atractylodes, siler, ginger

**zhi-dao-han*: inhibiting night sweating

HY-35 is based on the famous Jade Screen Formula. It nourishes *qi*, strengthens the body surface, and inhibits sweating. It is also helpful in preventing respiratory tract infections and has been found to have immuno-enhancing effects. Astragalus is the major herb and the primary *qi* tonic. Atractylodes strengthens the functioning of spleen and can help the major herb to promote the generation of *qi* and blood. Siler helps to eliminate external evils by coordinating with astragalus to dispel the evil without damage to *qi*. Siler also strengthens the body surface so that it can more effectively repel the external evil.

● Spleen and Liver Disharmony

Constitutional symptoms caused by disharmony of spleen and liver are mental and physical stress leading to anxiety, restlessness, nervousness, loss of appetite, depression, premenstrual tension, or menstrual irregularity. These symptoms are common in HIV (+) patients (especially females), and when they become the major complaints, the following formulas can be used.

HY-6 *he-jie** - I

> bupleurum, scute, pinellia, jujube,
> ginseng, licorice, ginger

HY-17 *he-jie* - II

> *tang-kuei*, peony, gardenia, ginger,
> atractylodes, hoelen, mentha,
> bupleurum, licorice, moutan

**he-jie*: harmonizing

HY-6 is based on Minor Bupleurum Combination. In Japan it is used as a immuno-regulating formula (Fujimaki 1989; Ono 1989) which is capable of increasing the number of T-4 and natural killer cells. The main ingredient of the formula is bupleurum, which nourishes the liver. When bupleurum and scute are combined, they have anti-inflammatory and detoxifying effects. Pinellia and ginger remove fluid accumulated in the stomach, relieve nausea, and promote appetite. A combination of ginseng, jujube and licorice is a stomachic and relieves the sensation of fullness beneath the heart.

HY-17 can be used for most emotional instabilities and is especially good for women's pre-menstrual syndrome. The principal herbs of this formula are bupleurum, *tang-kuei*, and peony. Bupleurum acts as an antipyretic stomachic agent for chest distention resulting from liver dysfunction. *Tang-kuei*, peony and moutan activate the blood and cool heat in the blood. Atractylodes and hoelen are stomachics and diuretics. Mentha helps to relieve depression. Ginger warms the body. Licorice coordinates the actions of the other herbs.

● Blood Stasis

Constitutional symptoms related to blood stasis and asthenic heat caused by blood stasis are purple or dark red tongue; fine, slow, and submerged pulse; congested sublingual vein; and blackish-striped fingernails. TCM holds that most long-term diseases must involve blood stasis, caused by both *qi* and blood deficiencies. The blood-generating suppressive side effects of AZT can also cause blood stasis. In PWAs, these symptoms exist together with anemia. TCM also holds that if one wants to tonify blood, the first step is to activate the stagnant blood. Therefore, if the patient has signs of anemia and also symptoms of blood stasis, the following formulas should first be used.

HY-12 *huo-xue** - I

> *tang-kuei*, rehmannia, peony, cnidium, coptis, scute, phellodendron, gardenia

---

HY-24 *huo-xue* - II

> *tang-kuei*, peony, rehmannia, persica, cnidium, carthamus

---

*huo-xue: activating the circulation of blood

HY-24 has a very strong effect in activating the circulation of blood and expelling stagnant blood. This formula is based on *Tang-kuei* Four Combination, the major blood-regulating formula. The addition of persica and carthamus strengthens the actions of *Tang-kuei* Four Combination.

HY-12 is even more effective than H-24 in treating asthenic heat caused by blood stasis and in promoting the circulation of blood. This formula is also based on *Tang-kuei* Four Combination with four cold and bitter herbs added. If long-term blood stasis is causing heat symptoms, this formula should be used.

● Energy Level, General Aches and Pains

Fatigue is a predominant complaint in HIV-infected patients and is caused by *qi* and *yang* deficiencies. The low energy level typical of this deficiencies causes a sensation of chill in the limbs. Influenza-like body aches are common symptoms which co-exist with fatigue and a sensation of heat inside the body. Since low energy level has detrimental effects, including loss of motivation and stamina, boosting the energy level is important both physiologically and psychologically. The following formulas can be used.

HY-36 *bu-yi** - I

> astragalus, ginseng, licorice, atractylodes, citrus rind, *tang-kuei*, cimicifuga, ginger, bupleurum, jujube

---

HY-37 *bu-yi* - II

> ginseng, astragalus, atractylodes, peony, hoelen, rehmannia, *tang-kuei*, cnidium, cinnamon, licorice

---

**bu-yi*: tonifying

Both formulas are based on well-known TCM tonification formulas. HY-36 is based on Ginseng and Astragalus Combination, the most important tonic for spleen, stomach, and the middle energizer. If spleen *qi* deficiency has been diagnosed and low energy is the major complaint, this formula should be used.

HY-37 is a tonic for *qi* and blood. If the patient manifests both *qi* and blood deficiencies, this formula is appropriate. It is a combination of the Four Major Herb Combination and *Tang-kuei* Four Combination. Cinnamon is added to warm the body and to tonify *yang*. Atractylodes is added to strengthen spleen and stomach functioning. If the patient feels very cold and has obvious symptoms of anemia, HY-28 can also be used (see Chapter 5).

Chronic body and muscle aches are other typical complaints in PWAs. The TCM conformation for this is *pi zheng* (a pathogenic blend of wind, cold, and dampness evils). A frequent complaint is a persistent influenza-like soreness throughout the body. In order to expel wind, dampness, and cold and promote blood circulation and the relief of pain, HY-38 should be employed.

HY-38 *qu-tong** - I

        salvia, red peony, moutan, persica, *chin-chiu*, cinnamon twigs, *tu-huo*, corydalis

---

**qu-tong*: pain-relieving

Clinical Evaluation of AIDS Therapies

Clinical observation is used to follow the course of the treatment and to determine whether the medication is efficacious. The practitioner monitors the subjective feelings of the patient, as well as any changes in the symptoms. The traditional tongue, tongue coating, pulse and complexion findings are also noted, as are such objective signs as body weight, severity of skin rash, and size of lymph nodes. This information is important for deciding whether to modify or discontinue the existing therapeutic measures. A well-designed recording chart should be prepared to record the clinical findings of every visit.

Clinical Follow-Up Records

Name:					
Date	Complaint	Symptoms	Tongue	Pulse	Treatments

In TCM practice, the above items are the most important to evaluate during each and every patient visit. This record can later be used for the clinical evaluation.

For Western evaluation of symptoms, use the following Karnovsky Score.

Karnovsky Score

100 – Normal
90 – Normal activity, minor symptoms
80 – Normal activity with effort, some symptoms
70 – Cares for self; unable to carry out normal activities
60 – Requires considerable assistance for most needs
50 – Requires considerable assistance & frequent care
40 – Disabled; requires special care & assistance
30 – Severely disabled; hospitalized, death not imminent
20 – Very sick; active supportive treatment needed
10 – Moribund; fatal processes rapidly progressing
0 – Dead

Laboratory Testing

One of the problems with research into AIDS therapies is the lack of laboratory tests which can reliably track the progress of the illness, thereby making it extremely difficult to know whether headway is being made with a seemingly promising therapy. Certainly treatment for some of the hallmark infections of AIDS can be evaluated, but the underlying immune deficiency is notoriously difficult to monitor (Barton 1989).

Despite this, several lab tests are somewhat useful for measuring the course of AIDS or ARC disorders. These test figures can serve as a crude index of the progression of the disease and as a guideline for selecting the appropriate herbal formulas.

● T-Cell Profile

The T-total count, T-4 count, T-8 count, and T-4/T-8 ratio are the figures most commonly used to show the body's level of immunity. But there is wide variability from measurement to measurement and from time to time, so one needs to establish a consistent trend in T-cell counts in order to establish confidence in their significance.

Serial measurement of T-4 (CD4) lymphocyte number in peripheral blood has a prognostic value. Creemers et al. found that decreases in immuno-functional responses were most frequent (83 - 100%) in individuals with a T-4 cell count of <400/ml, and were least frequent (3-21%) in subjects with a T-4 cell count of 600/ml. Frequency of decreased functional responses was intermediate in populations with 400-600/ml T-4 cells. The magnitude of functional responses differed significantly between groups with <400, 400-600, and >600 T-4 cells/ml, indicating that T-helper cell numbers decrease with a loss of immune function. A T-helper cell number of <400/ml in peripheral blood is a reliable indicator for the presence of moderate cellular immune dysfunction. Results support the concept that serial measurements of T-helper cell numbers are of prognostic value in HIV infection, provided the number of T-helper cells is <600/ml in peripheral blood. (Gupta 1986; Nicholson 1986; Creemers 1988).

In our experience, TCM immuno-enhancers have not produced an increase in the T-4 cells. More investigation is needed to find a proper formula for increasing T-4 cells per microliter, either by inhibiting the HIV or by enhancing the T-4 cell generating function.

● T-4/T-8 (CD4/CD8) Ratio

In AIDS or ARC, measurements of T-cells and the T-4/T-8 ratio are commonly used to monitor the progress of the disease and are usually included in a series of tests called the lymphocyte profile. T-4 helper cells experience a decline in PWAs, while T-8 suppressor cells generally increase early in the disease and decrease to normal levels later. As the disease progresses, the T-4/T-8 ratio declines. The ratio in normal persons is 1.8 to 2.3. For a moderately ill AIDS or ARC patient, the ratio ranges from 0.2 to 0.7, a level at which the patient can begin TCM therapies with every expectation of improving the ratio – sometimes to normal. The closer the ratio approaches 0.01, the more difficult it becomes for the reserve capacity of the immune system to rebound (Badgley 1986).

● P24

P24 is a measure of the level of production of HIV particles. It is presumed that the level of the P24 antigen in the serum roughly correlates with the level of viral replication in the body. Therefore, measurement of the P24 antigen level can help determine the effects of various treatments for HIV proliferation. In the AIDS Herbal Project, Dr. Keith Barton used this test to monitor the antiviral effects of the herbal formulas he prescribed (Barton 1989). The P24 antigen level is also predictive of the progression from HIV infection to full-blown AIDS; if the P24 antigen is detectable in the serum, there is a five-fold increased likelihood of developing AIDS within one year, as compared to a person with undetectable levels of P24 antigen levels.

We have used P24 levels in both our San Francisco and Lakewood clinical trials. In San Francisco, we affected a swing from a positive to a negative P24 level in one patient who was using AZT at the same time. In Lakewood, we affected a change from 170 to a negative level after three weeks of taking formula HY-31, without the semotenious use of AZT. Despite these successes, we need more cases from which to draw a conclusion.

● β-2-Microglobulin

This is a protein which is on the surface of lymphocytes. When the lymphocyte is damaged, the β-2-microglobulin is released into the blood stream and can be measured. It is an indicator of lymphocyte damage. A higher than normal level of this protein indicates an increased risk of AIDS development. A decreasing level of β-2-microglobulin may indicate improvement. This and the P24 are less expensive than the T-cell profile tests, but the T-cell profile remains the major index of the disease's progression.

The following tests are not so specific as the foregoing, but can also be used to evaluate the general condition of the patient's illness.

● ESR (erythrocyte sedimentation rate)

The sedimentation rate of red blood cells varies during the course of the disease. When it is elevated, the disease is progressing; if it approaches normal, the disease is tending to stabilize. The normal ESR range is 1 to 12.

● DHR (delayed type hypersensitivity reaction)

This test measures the immune system's ability to react to foreign antigens introduced into the skin. In AIDS or ARC patients, the immune system is often too weak to mount a reaction; this is called "anergy." The DHR test may be performed every four to six months to see whether the immune system has become stronger.

These lab tests can reflect the coping capacity of the patient's immune system to a certain degree and so can be used as a reference point for evaluating and monitoring our therapeutic measures.

It is not possible for TCM practitioners to order these lab tests on their own authority, and most of this information can only be obtained from the patient's Western physician. This situation makes it very difficult to use lab data to the best advantage.

In our first clinical trial, we found that the lab results did not always parallel the clinical symptoms. Some patients felt well, clinically, but their lab figures were declining; a few patients' lab results showed an increase of T-4 cells at the same time their subjective sense of well-being was deteriorating. For a clinical evaluation, it is crucial that the TCM practitioner consider all aspects of the patient's condition.

5

TCM Clinical Therapeutics for Complications of AIDS/ARC

Successful treatment of opportunistic infections and cancers in AIDS patients is a very important aspect of the whole therapeutic scheme, and recent breakthroughs in the treatment of PWAs have been primarily in this area.

Treatment of Opportunistic Infections

Protozoal Infections

● *Pneumocystis carinii* pneumonia (PCP)

Over 65% of all patients with AIDS will ultimately develop PCP, and each episode carries a 10 to 50% mortality rate. It is anticipated that, in 1991, 75,000 to 100,000 cases will occur. Thus it is appropriate to devote considerable attention to the prevention, diagnosis, and therapy of this protozoan process in an effort to decrease deaths. (Suffredini 1987). In AIDS patients, the signs and symptoms of the illness are frequently subtle, indistinct, and often dissociated from the lungs' histopathologic appearance. There is no reliable mechanism to determine drug sensitivities. Standard Western medical therapies are frequently associated with significant toxicities, limiting their long-term usefulness for the recurrent episodes of pneumonia common in AIDS patients.

The Western medical diagnosis of PCP is established by demonstrating the *P. carinii* organisms in stained pulmonary secretions or lung tissue. Its non-specific symptoms (fever, chills, cough, and shortness of breath) cannot be used as definite diagnostic criteria, but these symptoms can be used for TCM conformational diagnosis. Long clinical observation has yielded the empirical finding that AIDS patients with PCP tend to have a dull ashen complexion. These symptoms can be diagnosed as deficiency of both *qi* (vital energy) and lung *yin*. The purpose of treatment is to supplement *qi*, nourish *yin*, invigorate spleen and eliminate phlegm. The herbal formula which can be used is HY-7, a modification of Platycodon and Fritillaria Combination (*qing-fei-tang*), the ingredients of which are listed in Appendix 3.

HY-7 is designed to treat the pattern of symptoms (the conformation) and does not deal directly with the pathogen (the protozoa). Since *P. carinii* causes the interstitial pneumonia and the protozoa exist in the interstitial cells of the lungs, anti-protozoal herbs, most notably *Artemisia annua*, can be used to directly attack the parasite (see Chapter 7). *A. annua* has been used for many centuries as a treatment for fever and malaria, the latter in which protozoa exist in the red blood cells (Klayman 1985). Other herbs, such as *Dichroa febrifuga* (*chang-shan*), *Bupleurum chinense* (*chai-hu*), *Coptis chinensis* (*huang-lien*), and *Phellodendron amurense* (*huang-bo*) are frequently added to internally-used formulas.

PCP has been effectively treated by pentamidine isethionate and arrested by periodic use of aerosol pentamidine. TCM treatment can be used as an adjunctive measure to clear residual heat and phlegm of lung (Huichuan Zhang 1985). As soon as the PCP diagnosis is made, it is vital that the patient not delay conventional Western treatment. As a general rule for TCM practitioners in this country, advise the patient to first try any available conventional treatment for a disorder.

● Cryptosporidiosis

In AIDS, more than in any other immunodeficiency, cryptosporidiosis is likely to cause a persistent debilitating diarrhea (Masur 1985). Cryptosporidiosis has been reported in from 3 to 4% of AIDS patients in the United States. This is undoubtedly a conservative estimate, since not all AIDS patients are examined for the parasite (Soave 1987).

Watery diarrhea, cramping abdominal pain, weight loss, and flatulence are major symptoms. Most patients report exacerbation of diarrhea and abdominal cramps with food ingestion. Nausea, vomiting, myalgia, and malaise may also be present. Physical examination frequently reveals signs of dehydration. Patients may experience frequent (6-25 times) and voluminous (1-25 liters) daily bowel movements. These symptoms can persist for months.

Symptomatic of spleen and kidney deficiencies, these manifestations are treated by strengthening the functioning of the kidney and spleen. For this infection, however, internal treatment with orally administered herbal formulas sometimes is not strong enough to eliminate the pathogen. In this case, the formula can be administered as an enema to directly attack the pathogen.

The ordinal TCM treatments for diarrhea will be discussed later. To be presented here is a special method, anal administration of the protozoa-killing herbal formula. A modification of Anemone Combination, HY-27 contains the following in-gredients:

> anemone rhizome, coptis rhizome, *Fraxinus* bark,
> phellodendron, brucea fruit, dichroa root,
> *Sanguisorba* root, and *Terminalia chebula* fruit.

To administer, make a decoction of about 150 cc and keep it at room temperature. Infuse the decoction slowly into the rectum. The patient should stay in bed and keep the decoction in the rectum as long as possible. If this procedure can be done while the patient is sleeping, the effects will be better. Repeat two or three times.

Case #004 in our clinical study was a 42-year-old male PWA. His diarrhea had persisted for about 2 months. Every day he went to the bathroom about 20 times. The diarrhea was watery with undigested food, and he complained of ab-dominal and anal pain. He had lost more than 30 pounds and looked very tired; his complexion was lusterless. A lab test revealed oocytes of *Cryptosporidium* in his feces. At first, we treated him with herbal formulas for diarrhea administered orally (Pueraria, Coptis, and Scute Combination and Aconite, Ginseng, and Ginger Combination), but these had no positive effect on any of the symptoms. When the rectal administration formula, HY-27, was adopted, the diarrhea eventually stopped. He then gained weight, and his overall condition dramatically improved.

This case illustrates the importance of understanding the disease mechanism. Western medicine provided the necessary information about the pathogen, and with this information, the anally administered formula was used to directly attack the *Cryptosporidia* protozoa. Integrating the two medicines thus obtained better therapeutic results than either was able to achieve in isolation. Modern pharmacological research on the protozoa-killing properties of certain herbs is discussed in Chapter 7.

Fungal Infections

● Mucosal Candidiasis

Candida infection is a common occurrence in patients with AIDS. *Candida stomatitis* or *esophagitis* may be the initial manifestation of AIDS or may occur after Kaposi's sarcoma or another opportunistic process has been recognized (Masur 1985). Though candidiasis confined to the oropharynx is not considered sufficiently indicative of an underlying defect in cell-mediated immunity to establish a diagnosis of AIDS, the presence of *Candida esophagitis* in a previously healthy, un-medicated patient between the ages of 28 days and 60 years meets the Center for Disease Control's surveillance criteria for an AIDS diagnosis (Reichert 1985). In patients with AIDS/ARC, widespread visceral dissemination of *Candida* is infrequent, though the oral manifestation is common.

Clinically, *Candida stomatitis* is easy to diagnose. The thrush is characterized by whitish curd-like exudates on the dorsal or lateral tongue, or oropharynx, or buccal mucosa that can be easily scraped away with a cotton swab or tongue depressor. If *Candida* exists in the esophagus and gastrointes-tinal tract, there may be difficulty in swallowing and abdominal flatulence. Poor appetite, heartburn, and dyspepsia are also common complaints.

TCM considers this disease to be caused by asthenic heat emanating from spleen and heart. In AIDS/ARC patients with severe deficiencies in both *qi* and *yin*, the external evil can easily invade the body. There are two sub-types, one charac-terized by domination by external evil, the other by *qi* as-thenia.

Domination by external evil is defined by a short disease course; red, ulcerated tongue; oral mucosa covered with a cheese-like coating; mild pain; foul breath; yellowish tongue coating; and a fast pulse. Patients of this type are still in a fairly strong conformation. The principle of treatment is to clear away heat and detoxify and eliminate dampness.

Herbal formulas for this condition are Forsythia and Rhubarb Formula (*liang-ge-san*) and Rehmannia and Akebia Formula (*tao-chih-san*). For the *Candida esophagitis* infection in which the heartburn is the chief complaint, Coptis and Scute Combination is very effective.

We had one patient who suffered from heartburn for several weeks. Four hours after we administrated Coptis and Scute Combination, the burning sensation stopped, and after two weeks of treatment, this symptom never returned. (The ingredients of these formulas can be found in Appendix 3.)

Qi deficiency is defined by a long disease course, localized existence of the cheese-like coating, pale tongue, oral mucosa, deficient breath, a reluctance to speak, a sensation of heat in palms and soles, poor appetite, and a weak and fine pulse. Most AIDS/ARC patients with *Candida* belong to this type. The principle of treatment is to nourish and support *qi* and *yin*, and expel the toxin. One herbal formula which can be used is *Tang-kuei* and Cimicifuga Combination (*qing-re-bu-qi-tang*). An alternative is Clearing Heat and Nourishing *Yin* Formula. Its ingredients, as well as those of *qing-re-bu-qi-tang*, are listed in Appendix 3.

A decoction of this formula is to be divided into three portions to be taken each day.

For external treatment, clean the surface of the thrush with a decoction of licorice and coptis, then apply a powder made of indigo, mirabilitum, and Borneo camphor. This should be done after every meal and at bed time. Another method for topical treatment of oral *Candida* is to gargle with a decoction made of coptis rhizome, brucea rhizome, and licorice. This is a very bitter, but effective solution. We had three patients who had had oral *Candida* for years. After using this solution as a gargle for about one week, the *Candida* started to clear up. Dingqing Liu et al. reported that using an aerosol made from garlic extract cured two cases of lung candidiasis (Dingqing Liu 1986).

Viral Infections

● Herpes Virus Infections

Herpes zoster and *herpes simplex* infections occur with greater frequency in patients with AIDS/ARC than in the general population. For an HIV(+) patient, the occurrence of herpes zoster may signal the impending development of other AIDS/ARC-related diseases (Cockerell 1987). Patients with AIDS/ARC are often plagued by severe recurrent *herpes simplex* infections. These infections are often more extensive, longer-lasting, and less responsive to antiviral therapy with acyclovir than *herpes simplex* infections occurring in healthy hosts.

The skin lesions of *herpes simplex* and herpes zoster are painful, clustering in localized neurodermatomic sections. In AIDS/ARC patients, the most frequent areas of occurrence are the genital and perianal areas. Lesions looks like ulcerations and are red, painful, or itching. In our project, there were six patients who had developed these infections, four in the genital and groin area and two in the perianal and rectal area.

Traditional Chinese Medicine considers skin rashes to be a consequence of dampness-heat. Since the genital and perianal area are in the lower energizer and these areas are along the path of the liver meridian, herpes zoster and *herpes simplex* is a conformation of evils of dampness and heat blended to attack the lower energizer. The corresponding therapeutic approach is to clear away heat and eliminate dampness. This conformation can be further divided into heat-dominated or dampness-dominated types, the treatments for which are different.

If the patient has more heat symptoms, (fresh, red lesions; sharp pain; heat; a dry mouth; "flushing up"), HY-21, a modification of Gentiana Combination (*lung-tan-xie-gan-tang*), should be used. (Its ingredients are listed in Appendix 3.)

If the patient has more dampness symptoms, (dark lesions; dull pain; edema; a sticky, damp tongue coating), Magnolia and Hoelen Combination (*wei-ling-tang*) plus gentiana, gardenia, and scute should be used. (Ingredients listed in Appendix 3.)

Case #011 in our clinical study was an ARC male. He developed genital rashes in both groin areas which were fresh red and hot, with a pinching pain, and with more than 20 papules clustering together. Systemically, he had a low-grade fever with regular "flushing up" in the afternoons, classifying symptoms as those of the heat sub-type. After he had taken HY-21 for two weeks, the rashes faded, the pain subsided to itching, and the "flushing up" was reduced. Two weeks later, the rashes disappeared.

Case #033 was a 42-year-old ARC male who developed proctitis and perianal ulcers. He had diarrhea, averaging five bowel movements a day. He also felt pinched and hot, with "flushing up." After he had taken HY-21 for four weeks, the proctitis and ulcers were healed and the other symptoms reduced.

* Hepatitis B

Patients with AIDS commonly have clinical and histologic hepatic viral infections. Given the epidemiologic similarities of hepatitis B virus (HBV) and HIV infections, it is not surprising that markers of past HBV infection, namely hepatitis B surface antibody (anti-HBs) or hepatitis B core antibody (anti-HBc), are found in approximately 90% of AIDS patients (Lebovics et al. 1987). In our project, most patients had a history of HBV infections, and many of these had abnormal liver enzyme readings.

Clinical manifestations of hepatitis are anorexia, nausea, a sensation of fullness in the mid-abdominal region, dull pain in the liver area, and generalized weakness. In most cases, the liver is enlarged and tender. Liver function can be impaired to various degrees. According to clinical manifestations and pathologic changes, the disease is divided into two classes: icteric (marked by jaundice) and anicteric (without jaundice).

In TCM, acute icteric hepatitis is known as "jaundice of *yang* nature," and chronic persistent hepatitis or cirrhosis is known as "jaundice of *yin* nature." For anicteric hepatitis, TCM usually diagnoses stagnant liver *qi*. Most patients in our project were anicteric and had no obvious liver symptoms. Only one case developed obvious jaundice. The chronic clinical symptoms are so similar to those of general manifestations of AIDS/ARC and HIV infections that it is difficult to differentiate the liver problem through clinical investigation only. All the cases with liver problems in our project were discovered by lab tests of liver enzymic analysis.

The principle for treating anicteric or chronic hepatitis is to soothe the liver and invigorate stomach functioning. If there is abundant dampness, the first choice is to strengthen spleen functioning; if there is a deficiency of *qi* and *jing* (vital energy and vital essence, respectively), it is advisable to replenish vital essence and soothe the liver. Chronic hepatitis cases, like those in our project, can be divided into stagnation of liver *qi* and disharmony of the liver and spleen.

Liver *qi* stasis is common in anicteric hepatitis. Its manifestations are pain in the hypochondriac region, a sensation of fullness in the chest and stomach; nausea; belching; abdominal distention; anorexia; moderate fever; bitter taste in the mouth; thin, white tongue coating; and wiry pulse. For this type of hepatitis, the principle of treatment is to soothe the depressed liver and rectify the flow of its *qi* (vital energy). The herbal formula to be used is Bupleurum and Cypress Combination (*chia-hu-shu-gan-tang*), the ingredients of which are: bupleurum root, citrus fruit, white peony root, cypress rhizome, curcuma root, malia fruit, citrus rind, immature citrus fruit, and licorice root.

For cases with severe pain in the hypochondriac region, add corydalis rhizome, curcuma rhizome, and carthamus flower. For cases with anorexia and loose stools due to spleen deficiency, add white atractylodes and hoelen. For cases with irritability, bitter taste in the mouth, epistaxis, and rapid, wiry pulse, add gardenia fruit and moutan bark.

Disharmony of liver and spleen manifests distending pain or stinging located in the right hypochondriac region and is often aggravated by emotional disturbances or fatigue; a sensation of fullness in the stomach and abdomen; belching; anorexia; malaise; loose stools; concentrated urine; a thin, white, or slimy tongue coating; and a fine, taut pulse. The principle of treatment for this type is soothing the depressed liver and strengthening the functioning of the spleen and stomach. Bupleurum and Cypress Combination or Citrus and Pinellia Combination or both can be taken. (Ingredients are listed in Appendix 3.)

For patients with jaundice and high liver enzyme readings, HY-14 and HY-15 can be used. If the patient retains water, HY-15 should be used. To reduce the liver enzyme level (high SGPT and SGOT), schizandra should be added as a chief ingredient.

Bacterial Infections

● Tuberculosis

Although tuberculosis is not considered an opportunistic infection, a high incidence of tuberculosis has been found among AIDS/ARC patients. Between 1981 and 1984, 5.4% of all reported New York City AIDS patients had tuberculosis (Duncanson et al. 1987), 80% of these in disseminated form.

The typical symptoms of disseminated tuberculosis are asthenic fever, facial "flushing up," night sweating, chills, anorexia, and weight loss. Since pulmonary tuberculosis is not so common, coughing and shortness of breath are not predominant symptoms. Patients usually have a red or dark red tongue and a fast, fine pulse. Conformational diagnosis of this condition is fever due to asthenia of the five solid organs, i.e. a severe *yin* deficiency of all organs. The principle of treatment is to nourish *yin* and clear away heat.

Herbs which can be used to treat low-grade fever are artemisia (*qing-hao*) and lycium bark (*di-gu-pi*). Herbs for night sweating are schizandra fruit (*wu-wei-zi*), *Tritici* grain (*fu-xiao-me*), *Nelumbo* seed (*lian-zi*), and *Oryza* root (*ru-tou-gan*) (Xiangjun Chen 1987). Herbal formulas we have used in clinical trials and which obtained good results in eliminating low-grade fever and night sweating, as well as improving general health, are HY-18, a modification of *Chin-chiu* and Tortoise Shell Formula, and HY-39. (Ingredients are listed in Appendix 3.)

● *Mycobacterium Avium-Intracellulara* Infections (MAI)

With the increasing incidence of AIDS, disseminated MAI infection has become more and more common. Autopsy findings at Memorial Sloan-Kettering Cancer Center of New York revealed disseminated MAI infection in more than 60% of its AIDS patients (Klein 1987). Its pathogenesis and pathology somewhat resemble those of tuberculosis, as does its clinical manifestations.

Persistent fever, diarrhea, night sweating, and weight loss appear to be the most common symptoms. A watery, non-bloody diarrhea differentiates MAI from tuberculosis. In conventional Western medicine, an infection in patients without AIDS is treated with anti-tuberculosis drugs, but for patients with AIDS, those treatments are not very effective. However, since the clinical manifestations are similar in both cases, the conformational diagnostic and treatment methods are also similar.

Opportunistic Cancers

Western medicine employs three basic methods for treating malignant tumors: surgery, radiotherapy, and chemotherapy. In AIDS patients, malignant tumors usually are not localized, thus making surgery very difficult to perform. Some patients try corrosive injections under the base of the Kaposi's sarcoma lesions, but this method can't be used for visceral KS lesions, and possible side effects are not known.

Radiotherapy for KS and other AIDS-related malignancies has achieved therapeutic responses, but radiation is a non-specific cell-killer and immuno-suppressor. For patients with pre-existing immunodeficiency, this therapy is far from ideal.

Chemotherapy uses chemically pure drugs to control or destroy cancer cells. Most of them are cytotoxics and tend to damage healthy cells as well. They are also immuno-suppressors. The toxic build-up debilitates the body's strength and can hasten the progress of the malignancy. Malignancies in AIDS patients are one of the most contradictory and difficult conditions to treat in Western medicine.

Chinese medicine has a different approach (Hsu 1982; Situ 1987). While Western medicine adopts allopathic procedures to kill cancer cells directly, and TCM also employs "toxins to attack toxins," this method is by no means a major principle of the treatment espoused in classic Chinese medical texts. When cancer invades the body, it naturally generates resistance, and TCM aims to strengthen this resistance so that the body can eliminate the cancer on its own. In AIDS patients, though, this ability has been badly damaged by the HIV virus. The method which TCM uses to strengthen the body's capacity for resistance is called *fuzheng*.

In China, the treatment of tumors by means of an integration of TCM and Western therapies has been studied and clinically tested for more than twenty years. In treating third-stage stomach cancer by combining chemotherapy with TCM therapies, the five-year survival rate is 46-52%, as compared to 11-33% with chemotherapy alone (editorials in *Chinese Journal of Integrated Traditional and Western Medicine* 1987; Lapp 1987). Improved results also have been obtained in liver, lung, breast, and nasopharyngeal cancers and leukemia.

* *Fuzheng* Cancer Therapy

Fuzheng has several meanings that apply to the treatment of malignancies. It enhances the immunity of the body in order to enable it to eliminate the cancer cells. It supports the patient's general health, making the body more able to tolerate the toxic effects of the cancer-metabolic products and the radiation and chemical treatments, and it treats specific side effects of radiotherapies and chemotherapies (nausea, vomiting, suppression of blood-generating functions) (Daizhao Zhang 1988). Therefore, combining Western methods with *fuzheng* therapy makes it possible to increase the dose and duration of Western therapies, and thereby intensify therapeutic effects.

Two *fuzheng* formulas have been used by the Cancer Institute and the Hospital of the Chinese Academy of Medical Sciences in Beijing (Yan Sun et al. 1987). FZ #2 is chiefly a kidney tonic, but also contains blood and *qi* tonics; it is used for general cancer patients. The ingredients are astragalus root 30g, ligustrum fruit 15g, *tang-kuei* 15g, *Millettia reliculata* 15g, lycium fruit 15g, and citrus rind 6g. FZ #4 is a kidney tonic, used for cancer patients with a severe kidney deficiency. The ingredients of the formula are astragalus root 30g, ligustrum fruit 15g, *Millettia reliculata* 15g, polygonatum rhizome 15g, and cuscuta seed 15g. These formulas were given to cancer patients during their conventional radio- or chemotherapies.

Long-term follow-up has indicated very encouraging results. Since 1974, clinical trials have been carried out, using *fuzheng* herbs either alone or as adjuvant therapy during radiotherapy or chemotherapy. A 10-year follow-up study of 213 cancer patients treated with *fuzheng* formulas found that, in 50 patients who received *fuzheng* therapy during remission, 44 were still alive, while in the control group, only 13 out of 21 survived (p<0.05). In three random studies, 32 of 43 patients with cervical and breast carcinoma treated by radiation and *fuzheng* therapy survived, but only 23 out of 46 patients who received radiation alone survived (p<0.5). Of 44 patients who received *fuzheng* therapy and chemotherapy, 24 are alive today, though this difference was insignificant as compared with the control group (Yan Sun et al. 1987).

The follow-up study also showed a correlation between the improvement of non-specific cell-mediated immunity and long-term survival. The possibility of improving the chances for long-term survival by adequate use of *fuzheng* therapy may exist because of these herbs' immuno-regulating functions, especially if they can stimulate the production of interferon and eliminate excess immuno-suppressor cells. (The pharmacological effects of *fuzheng* will be discussed in Chapter 7.)

● Kaposi's Sarcoma (KS)

Since the outbreak of the AIDS epidemic, over 16,000 cases of this disorder have been reported in the United States. The incidence of KS is approximately 30% among homosexual patients with AIDS, while it is less than 5% among intravenous drug-using AIDS patients (Hymes 1987). The cases have occurred in persons aged 19 to 64, with the mean age being 37.7. Approximately 48% of all homosexual males with AIDS at present have or will eventually develop KS during the course of their illness, whereas 41% contract PCP and another 13% develop other opportunistic infections (Krigel 1985). Eight of our ten AIDS patients in SFAAHP manifested Kaposi's sarcoma.

KS lesions are located on the skin or in different internal organs. The skin lesions are pink, purple or brown in color, and highly pigmented in black patients. The common location for these lesions is in the extremities. Lesions of the mucosa, especially in the mouth or upper palate, may be a clue to lesions in internal organs. These are firm, unblanched, and fixed to the underlying subcutaneous tissue. Skin lesions generally are asymptomatic, with no itching, pain, or bleeding. Mucous membrane involvement in the mouth and in the esophagus can cause difficulty in swallowing. Internally, lesions may occur in the gastrointestinal tract, lungs, spleen, heart, lymph nodes, and any organ with endothelium tissue. A positive diagnosis can be established by a biopsy.

Besides local lesions, AIDS patients with KS may have systemic symptoms (dull, ashen complexion; fatigue; low energy; poor appetite; loss of vocal power; pale tongue with teeth marks; purple spots or pigmentation on the tongue with a white, thin coating; congested sublingual vein; fine, weak pulse; and dark pigmentation in fingernails and toenails). On the basis of these symptoms, together with the local lesions, the TCM diagnosis is blood stasis due to *qi* deficiency and blocking of the meridians. The principle of treatment is to activate blood circulation, remove stagnant blood, clean the collateral meridians, and disperse masses. We have been using formulas HY-19 and HY-5 (modifications of Forsythia and Laminaria Combination and *Lithospermum* and Oyster Shell Combination, respectively) combined with *fuzheng* (immuno-enhancing) and *quxie* (antiviral) treatments for SFAAHP patients with Kaposi's sarcoma. (Ingredients of these two formulas are found in Appendix 3.)

● Non-Hodgkin's Lymphomas and Hodgkin's Disease

Non-Hodgkin's lymphomas are a frequent manifestation of AIDS. These tumors may or may not be confined to the brain. Primary brain lymphomas are associated with an extremely poor prognosis. Hodgkin's disease is also seen in patients at risk for AIDS. Advanced (stage IV) disease appears to be more frequent in these patients. There is as yet no ideal standard therapy for patients with an AIDS-related tumor. This information will require much more experimental data (Ahmed 1987).

From the TCM point of view, the clinical manifestations of these tumors are similar to those of leukemia. According to TCM, etiologically, they are caused by long-hidden and undeveloped toxins (external evils). Their conformations (symptom complexes) mostly belong to deficiency of *yin*, asthenic fire and the accumulation of phlegm. The treatment principles for these conditions are nourishing *yin*, especially kidney *yin*, softening the hard lumps, and dispelling the nodes (Qiyuan Sun 1989). We have been using this principle to treat patients with these complications.

Other Common Complications of AIDS/ARC

● Anemia

A longitudinal study found that higher initial leukocyte and lymphocyte counts were directly correlated with survival at two years. In this study, 55% of the patients with a normal number of lymphocytes at presentation were alive after two years, in contrast to only 30% of the patients with low lymphocyte counts (Safai et al. 1985). It is obvious that keeping the WBC and lymphocyte counts at a high level is important in prolonging the patient's life.

Leukopenia and lymphopenia are prominent laboratory findings in AIDS/ARC and HIV (+) persons. In our patient groups, the average white blood cell counts were 3,850 (AIDS), 4,183 (ARC), and 2,492 (HIV+) respectively. All are much lower than the normal count of 6,100. In a group of patients who were not HIV-infected, the average WBC count was 6,333. The figures for lymphocytes in the same groups were 1,188, 1,471, and 1,233, respectively. The figure of the non-HIV infection control group was 1,965. The normal figure is 2,363. Although the patient groups were not very large and our results may be due to the size of our sample, the average WBC and lymphocyte counts are still illustrative.

In addition to WBC and lymphocyte counts abnormalities, red blood cell counts of AIDS/ARC and HIV(+) patients are also much lower than normal. The average numbers for RBC counts for AIDS, ARC, and HIV(+) patients in our project were 4.14, 3.88, and 4.68, respectively. The normal range for this figure is 4.7 - 6.1, as are the hemoglobin and HCT. These figures suggest that the all blood-cell-generating functions have been suppressed in AIDS/ARC and HIV(+) patients.

Among AIDS/ARC patients of SFAAHP, the subgroup taking AZT treatment had even more severe anemic symptoms. The WBC, lymphocyte, and RBC counts for this group were 3050, 812, and 3.29, respectively. Such patients require regular blood transfusions when their blood counts drop too low, and, frequently, AZT therapy has to be interrupted.

Clinically, patients with anemia show typical TCM symptoms indicating deficiency in blood and *qi*: pale, lusterless complexion; rough and dry skin; chills; cold limbs; pale tongue; fast, fine, and weak pulse. For a long-term illness like AIDS/ARC, these symptoms usually co-exist with blood stasis, manifested in such symptoms as a swarthy, "dirty" complexion, blue-purple or pigmented tongue, and congested sublingual vein. Two of our most severe blood stasis and anemic patients had dark-striped fingernails.

The conformation of anemia in AIDS/ARC patients is blood deficiency and stasis. The principle of treatment for this condition is first to activate blood and expel stagnant blood, then to tonify blood. Tonifying the kidney is also important, because TCM holds that bone marrow is under the control of kidney, and only by strengthening the kidney can the manufacture of bone marrow be stimulated. Two other organs, the liver and spleen, should also be tonified. Liver is the organ in TCM which generates blood, and spleen is the organ which regulates the circulation of blood (Qingcai Zhang 1988).

If there are symptoms of blood stasis, the first measure for treating anemia is to use blood-activating and stasis-expelling herbal formulas. In our project, HY-24, the blood-activating formula (for ingredients see Appendix 3) was used, and found to be effective. After 2-4 weeks of taking this formula, patients' complexions regained their luster, tongue color became more red and sublingual vein congestion was reduced.

After the blood stasis has been reduced, the blood tonification formula, HY-23, can be used. (Its ingredients are listed in Appendix 3.)

Patients with extremely low blood counts, chills, and a very low energy level may benefit from (young) deerhorn, which is very effective in combination with certain blood-activating and heat-reducing herbs. In our project, we used it in a combination coded HY-28. Patients took one gram twice a day. The effects were obvious: one AIDS patient was able to go back to part-time work, feeling energetic enough to do manual labor. Another patient had been troubled by persistent chills and was totally lacking in motivation, yet began to feel warm and chat with people after two weeks.

In order to treat leukopenia caused by viral infection, or radio- or chemotherapy, much clinical and experimental research has been done in China. The reports which follow have shown effective results and their methods can be used for treatment of leukopenia in AIDS patients.

Twenty-two patients with leukopenia and *qi* deficiency who were unresponsive to conventional Western treatment were treated with an infusion made of the leaf of *Epimedium sagittatum*, 15 grams per pack. The dosage was three packs daily for the first week, then reduced to two packs daily till the end of the therapeutic course (30-45 days). Of the 14 patients who complied with the treatment regimen, three were cured, four were markedly improved (increased WBC by at least 1,500), and five were significantly improved (increased WBC by at least 1,000). Leukocyte count was increased from 2440±992 to 4060±966. The immune-complex titers, and serum $Zn++$ and $Mg++$ were decreased. The lymphocyte transformation rate was increased from 269±123 to 391±154 (Fuchun Liu 1985).

AZT-induced leukopenia is similar to chemotherapy-induced leukopenia. Thirty-seven cases of chemotherapy-induced leukopenia were treated with a tablet (50mg each) of ginsenosides (an active component of ginseng) at 50-100 mg, two to three times daily for a total dose of 1.6-6.8 grams. The treatment increased the WBC count to above 4000 within 2 weeks in 82% of the patients. No side effects were observed (Jichang Zhou 1987).

Shengbai (raising leukocyte count) Tablet is made of the following herbs: *Psoralea*, epimedium, placenta, ligustrum, cornus, astragalus, jujube, *tang-kuei*, salvia, spatholubus, notoginseng, and *Polygonum*. It was used in the treatment of chemotherapy-induced leukopenia at a dosage of five tablets thrice daily. After 2 weeks of treatment (concurrent with chemotherapy), 26 patients (56.5%) had their WBC count increased by 1.5 million/ml and 18 (39.1%) had it increased by 1-1.5 million/ml. The total effective rate was 95.6%. The therapeutic result was stable (Jinyuan Wang 1988).

This treatment (blood -activating and -tonifying) has obtained good results. Subjectively, the sensation of chill in the limbs was reduced and the energy level improved. Objectively, the patients' complexions regained their former luster, and tongue color turned red or lost its pigment. The lab tests showed improvement in WBC, RBC, and lymphocyte counts (see Table 5-1).

Table 5-1 Blood Counts

Group	WBC		Lymphocyte		RBC	
	Before	After	Before	After	Before	After
AIDS	3966	4014	1099	1138.7	3.87	3.96
AIDS + AZT	3050	3050	812	765	3.29	3.04
ARC	4183	4950	1471	1457.6	3.88	4.41
HIV(+)	3785	3814	1233	1219.5	4.68	4.83
EBV	6333	6320	1965	2136	4.22	4.32
Normal	6100		2363		4.7 - 6.1	

Case #007 was a 32-year-old male PWA. When he joined the project, he had encephalitis diagnosed by CAT scan and CF analysis, which was accompanied by headaches, loss of balance, lymphadenopathy, and skin lesions. He was chronically depressed, his complexion was pale and without luster, his tongue pale with obvious teeth marks, and his fingernails black-striped. He felt constantly chilled and without motivation. His blood counts were very low (WBC 3,000, HCT 27.8). His TCM diagnosis was extreme deficiency of *qi*, blood and heart, confused by phlegm. After approximately three weeks on HY-23 and HY-28, his blood counts improved (WBC 4,100, HCT 29.5). He became much more talkative, and no longer felt chilled. The black stripes on his fingernails began to fade and his face regained it former luster.

● Diarrhea

Diarrhea with profound emaciation is a major AIDS symptom. Intestinal disease may be observed in 50-60% of patients with AIDS in the United States and close to 100% of AIDS patients in Africa and Haiti (Soave 1987). Persistent diarrhea, lasting longer than one week, may lead to severe dehydration and the loss of essential body salts. Because of the underlying immunodeficiency, AIDS/ARC and HIV (+) patients tend to have frequent diarrhea caused by inadequate food intake (resulting in acute gastritis) or protozoan infection. The HIV can also infect colon cells directly and cause diarrhea (Kolata 1988).

The symptoms of gastritis, amebiasis, and giardiasis vary, but most patients have watery, foul-smelling diarrhea, abdominal distention, and flatulence. In its acute stage, there are cramps in the lower abdomen, fever, and bloody diarrhea. In TCM these symptoms are attributed to deficiency of the middle energizer and dysfunction of spleen and stomach. If the diarrhea becomes persistent, with undigested food, and is watery and odorless, kidney deficiency is also a contributing factor (Qieliang Fu 1985).

TCM regards the spleen and stomach as the postnatal sources of vitality. When treating any disease, regulating the functions of the spleen and stomach is the first step in enabling the patient's body to improve its condition. This is also true for AIDS/ARC patients who have diarrhea. Especially in extreme deficiencies like AIDS, tonification is the basic principle of TCM treatment. However, TCM theory also holds that, if the patient is in a very weak or severely deficient condition, nutritive and tonifying measures will not be effective until such spleen and stomach problems as diarrhea or gastrointestinal dysfunction are resolved.

If the diarrhea is acute, with symptoms of gastritis, such as fever, lower abdominal cramps, and bloody stools, stomach dampness and heat is the TCM diagnosis. The herbal formula to be used is HY-9, a modification of Pueraria, Coptis, and Scute Combination (ingredients listed in Appendix 3). To augment this formula, two additional formulas can be used. If fever and heat are dominant in the patient's conformation, Agastache Formula should be added; if not, use Ginseng and Atractylodes Formula (ingredients listed in Appendix 3).

If the diarrhea has already become chronic, with a cold pain which can be relieved by pressing or warming the abdomen, and if the diarrhea is watery and odorless, with undigested food, it is because of extreme deficiency of spleen and stomach. If the patient feels cold pain in his or her lower abdomen, hot sensation in the upper body, cold in the lower body, and chill in the limbs, HY-25 can be used. In its most severe form, kidney deficiency also plays an important role. In this case, HY-20, a modification of Aconite, Ginseng, and Ginger Combination should be used.

In some persistent diarrhea cases, especially those due to amebiasis and giardiasis, these methods may not be effective. If the diarrhea persists, and amebiasis or giardiasis has been diagnosed, the parasiticide HY-26, a modification of Anemone Combination, can be administered to directly attack the parasites. (Ingredients of these formulas are listed in Appendix 3.)

6

Comprehensive TCM Therapeutic Measures

Herbal formulas are central to Traditional Chinese Medicine, but they are not the only TCM therapeutic measures available to AIDS/ARC patients. In the holistic approach characteristic of TCM, acupuncture, manipulation, and *qi gong* (breathing exercises) have all been used in treating AIDS/ARC, with especially beneficial effects in relieving symptoms and improving the quality of life.

Acupuncture

A natural means of stimulation without the use of pharmaceuticals, acupuncture is easy to perform, and the beneficial effects can be seen immediately after each treatment.

Here we will discuss only the principles and clinical applications of acupuncture in treating AIDS/ARC and HIV (+) patients.

Prescribing the Points

There are two ways of selecting acupuncture points: the local points (the *ahshi* or "ouch" points and the points near the disordered area) and the points along the pathway of the meridian.

Ahshi points are found by locating tenderness or pain at the site of greatest sensitivity: "Where there is a pain, there lies a point." This method has not been used frequently in AIDS/ARC treatment. Since HIV infection is a systemic syndrome, local tender spots do not always exist. Where such areas do exist, of course, this method can be used.

The selection of points along the meridian pathways essentially determines the prescription principle of acupuncture. According to the *jingluo* theory ("where the meridian passes, there is healing"), the appropriate meridian first must be chosen, then the appropriate points along this meridian and finally the prescription of specific points. The proper meridians are those in which the related organs have been affected by AIDS/ARC pathogenic processes. As was indicated in Chapters 2 and 3, most AIDS/ARC patients show kidney, spleen, and lung deficiencies; therefore, it is these three channels and their collateral channels which most frequently are chosen. From these related channels, the specific appropriate points are selected.

In addition to body points, ear points are effective for conditioning body functions. Ear points are chosen according to TCM theory concerning their correspondence to the organs. For example, for kidney deficiency, the kidney point on the ear should be stimulated. Besides these corresponding points, the *shenmen* and endocrine points generally are used for strengthening bodily health and conditioning energy (Smith 1989).

Clinical Methodology

In the practice followed by SFAAHP, acupuncture therapies chiefly were conducted by Dr. Misha Cohen and her colleagues of *Quan Yin* Acupuncture and Herb Center of San Francisco. She has been treating AIDS/ARC patients with acupuncture for more than five years with encouraging results (Misha Cohen 1986). The following discussion is based on her findings.

The differential diagnosis discussed in previous chapters is useful in determining the therapeutic strategy for formulating the prescription of points. To summarize the symptoms of AIDS/ARC patients in order to diagnose the conformation, or symptom pattern, is the first step of acupuncture treatment. For these conformations, appropriate acupuncture treatments already have been formulated.

AIDS/ARC patients have shown various symptoms which are signs of deficiency, particularly as kidney, spleen, and lung deficiencies. At the AIDS stage, patients will show more symptoms of deficient heat, toxic heat, blood stagnation, and *shen* disturbances.

Moxibustion is a method used in acupuncture practice. It involves the application of an ignited cone or stick of mugwort over the acupuncture points in order to stimulate the body through heat. Moxibustion is primarily used for asthenic conditions.

The following procedures indicate acupuncture and moxibustion treatments for AIDS/ARC according to this kind of differential diagnosis (Misha Cohen 1986) used in the SFAAHP project.

Basic Acupuncture Treatment

The following treatment uses moxibustion only (for deficiency); other treatment includes acupuncture. The points used are:

S 36 (*zusanli*): Tonify *qi* and strengthen deficiencies by replenishing middle energizer, regulating the stomach and strengthening the spleen, clearing the channels, invigorating the collateral channels, and improving general health. Insertion 1.0 - 1.5 cun, 10-20 minutes with moxa roll.

G 39 (*xuanzhong*): Strengthen marrow and blood. Insertion 1.0 - 1.5 cun, 5-15 minutes with moxa roll.

Cv 6 (*qihai*): Strengthen *qi* and kidney by reinforcing *yang* and *jing* (vital essence), impelling the upward flow of *yang*, and reinforcing *qi*. Insertion 1.0 - 2.0 cun, 10-20 minutes with moxa roll.

Cv 8 (*shenque*): Restore *yang* energy by strengthening spleen and regulating stomach, warming *yang*, and recovering prostration, 5-15 minutes with moxa roll, no needling. (This is contraindicated for patients with heat-type constitutions.)

B 43 (*gaohuang*): Strengthen deficient conditions by enhancing the functioning of *qi*, reinforcing kidney, strengthening spleen, regulating stomach, and calming heat and spirit. Insertion 0.3 - 0.5 cun, 10-20 minutes with moxa roll.

For spleen *qi* deficiency together with blood deficiency, add the following to the basic treatment:

Cv 12 (*zhongwan*): Strengthen stomach and spleen by reducing nausea, regulating stomach and reversing the adverse flow of *qi*, strengthening spleen and dissipating dampness. Insertion 1.0-2.0 cun, 10-20 minutes with moxa roll.

Sp 6 (*sanyinjiao*): Strengthen spleen by eliminating dampness, tonifying blood, invigorating spleen and stomach, and sedating the mind. Insertion 1.0-1.5 cun, 10-20 minutes with moxa roll.

B 20 (*pishu*): Strengthen spleen by dissipating pathogenic dampness, regulating stomach, and reversing the adverse flow of stomach *qi*. Insertion 0.3-0.6 cun, 5- 20 minutes with moxa roll.

B 21 (*weishu*): Strengthen stomach and spleen by dispelling pathogenic dampness and dissolving intestinal stasis. Insertion 0.3-0.6 cun, 5-15 minutes with moxa roll.

For kidney *jing* (essence) deficiency, add the following to the basic treatment:

K 3 (*taixi*): Strengthen kidney and sperm by nourishing the liver and the kidney, regulating the *chong* and *ren* channels, clearing lung of pathogenic heat and sedating cough. Insertion 1.0-1.5 cun, 5-10 minutes with moxa roll.

B 23 (*shenshu*): Moxa is particularly important here in order to strengthen kidney, nourish *yin*, and strengthen *yang*, the brain and marrow, increase the activities of the brain and improve vision. Insertion 0.5-1.0 cun, 1-15 minutes with moxa roll.

For kidney *yin* deficiency, add the following to the basic treatment:

K 3 (*taixi*): See above.

K 7 (*fuliu*): Tonify kidney by inhibiting sweating, regulating the fluid system, and dissipating pathogenic dampness. Insertion 1.0-1.5, 5-10 minutes with moxa roll.

B 23 (*shenshu*): See above.

H 6 (*yinxi*): Inhibiting sweating, regulating heart and the mind, clearing pathogenic blood heat, cooling blood, and relaxing the chest. Insertion 0.2-0.4 cun, 10-15 minutes with moxa roll.

For kidney *yang* deficiency, use moxibustion when using the following points:

B 23 (*shenshu*): See above.

Gv 4 (*mingmen*): Strengthen kidney *yang* by replenishing *yuan qi*, reinforcing *jing* (vital essence) and strengthening *yang*. Insertion 0.5-1.0 cun, 5-15 minutes with moxa roll.

C 4 (*guanyuan*): Strengthen kidney *yang* by reinforcing *yuan qi*, reviving *yang*, rescuing the collapse of *yin* and *yang*, and encouraging the flow of *qi* and blood. Insertion 1.0-2.0 cun, 10-20 minutes with moxa roll.

Cv 6 (*qihai*): See above.

For lung *qi* and lung *yin* deficiencies, add the following to the basic treatment:

L 7 (*lieque*): Open and strengthen lung by dissipating wind, clearing exterior symptoms, and invigorating the collaterals. Insertion 0.5-0.8 cun, 5-10 minutes with moxa roll.

LI 4 (*hegu*): Relieve exterior evils by dissipating pathogenic heat, sedating pain, and regulating *qi* and blood. Insertion 1.0 cun, 5-10 minutes with moxa roll.

B 13 (*feishu*): Strengthen lung by dissipating pathogenic wind and heat, ventilating lung, encouraging the flow of *qi*, nourishing *yin*, and dissipating pathogenic heat. Insertion 0.5-1.0 cun, 10-20 minutes with moxa roll.

Pain

The "four gates for pain" are LI 4 (*hegu*), left and right, and LI 3 (*sanjian*), left and right. Insertion 0.5-0.8 cun, 3-5 minutes with moxa roll.

Sore Throat and Swollen Glands

A traditional combination for treating sore throat and swollen glands is K 6 (*zhaohai*): insertion 0.3-0.5 cun, 5-10 minutes with moxa roll together with L 7 (*Lieque*).

For disturbance of *shen*, add the following to the basic treatment:

H 7 (*shenmen*): Pacify spirit and calm heart by regulating and sedating heart and mind. Insertion 02-0.3 cun, 10-15 minutes with moxa roll.

H 6 (*yinxi*): See above.

Sishencong (extraordinary points): Pacify spirit and strengthen the brain. Used for migraine, dizziness, epilepsy, mania, and hydrocephalus. Insertion 0.5-1.0 cun, 5-10 minutes with moxa roll.

The following spirit (*shen*) points are helpful:

K 24 (*lingxu*) insertion 0.2-0.4 cun, 5-10 minutes with moxa roll.

K 25 (*shencang*) insertion 0.2-0.4 cun, 5-10 minutes with moxa roll.

Schedules for Acupuncture Treatment

Usually the patient is treated once a week with acupuncture; however, if time and finances allow, treatments twice a week are recommended. During each treatment, the needles should be kept in the body about 20 minutes. The time of application of moxa roll is dependent on the points used.

Sterilization and Acupuncturist Safety

The HIV virus is very heat-sensitive and, therefore, much easier to eliminate than the hepatitis B virus (Shanahan 1985). Subjecting any suspect object or material to 56° C for 30 minutes will eliminate any risk. Boiling for 10 minutes is also adequate. Any spillage of suspect material can be rendered safe by the application of household bleach. In laboratories, 10% hydrochloride solution soak is regarded as adequate to decontaminate surfaces.

Acupuncture needles can be sterilized in a high-temperature and high-pressure sterilizer, but for absolute safety, disposable needles always should be used. Each needle should be used on only one patient, and sterilized before it is disposed.

It is safe for the hands and fingers of the acupuncturist to touch the skin of patients in order to locate acupuncture points, provided there are no cuts or abrasions in those areas or on the fingers of the acupuncturist. One can safely "seal" an acupuncture point in a suspected AIDS patient with the bare finger without fear of contracting the virus, so long as the skin is absolutely unbroken at the point of contact.

Results of Acupuncture Treatments

The generalized principle for choosing acupuncture points has been described, however, every patient requires his or her own prescription. When Dr. Michael Smith evaluated the results of acupuncture treatment in the Lincoln Hospital Acupuncture Clinic, Bronx, New York, he found that individualized and variable treatment according to the patients' symptoms produced better therapeutic results. Also diagnostic indications vary from visit to visit, even for the same patient (Smith 1989).

Short-Term Benefits

An increased energy level and an improved sense of well-being, as well as the alleviation of abnormal sweating and diarrhea, can be seen after just a few treatments. Some patients gain weight and recover enough energy to return to work. These short-term improvements are encouraging.

Long-Term Benefits

Smith reported that, in his patient group, the survival rate of patients treated with acupuncture is much higher than the average for ARC or AIDS patients. In his early patient group, there were 14 with ARC. Among them, five were not followed up. Of the other nine patients, five were still living when the study concluded in 1987.

Among Smith's early AIDS patient group treated with acupuncture, one man diagnosed with KS in 1981 reported that the acupuncture reduced the side effects of chemotherapy, helped him sleep more comfortably and improved his energy level. He continued to receive acupuncture massages in the following years and was identified as one of the longest AIDS survivors on record at the time of his death in 1987.

About 40% of Smith's initial AIDS patients were doing well during his early acupuncture and herbal treatments in 1982 and 1983. He is very optimistic about TCM treatment for AIDS/ARC, observing that "now that our diagnostic skill and herbal capabilities have improved, one might hope for more significant results in the future."

Manipulations and Massotherapies

Manipulation for AIDS

Manipulation, massage, and varieties of body work have been used in many alternative healing clinics for AIDS/ARC and HIV (+) patients to improve the general health of the patient and relieve symptoms.

Chinese manipulative therapy has various therapeutic effects, among them clearing meridian passageways through massage of the channel path, regulating the circulation of blood and *qi*, expelling wind and cold evils, and relieving muscular spasms, pain, and stress. It is not limited to disorders of the spinal column and limbs, but treats the whole body. It can also heal internal diseases. In short, manipulation is a passive way to relax the body, both physically and mentally.

As has been noted, AIDS/ARC patients have common symptoms of kidney deficiency: a tendency to have lower back pain, lassitude in the loins and legs, and body aches. These symptoms can be easily relieved by manipulation. For patients with spleen deficiency, spleen- and stomach-strengthening massage methods can be helpful in regulating gastrointestinal functioning. Anxiety and mental stress are also common symptoms in AIDS/ARC patients, and manipulation brings relief through relaxation.

Methods of Manipulation

There are eight basic manipulation methods: pressing, rubbing, stroking, pinching, rolling, digging, kneading, and vibrating (or turning). Physicians often combine them when working with different areas of the body. Effectiveness of manipulation depends to a great extent on the manipulator's expertise. For best results, the manipulator should have certain basic training (*kung fu* for example) to strengthen the muscles needed for manipulation. The methods can be learned only by apprenticeship to an experienced practitioner.

Manipulation also uses the acupuncture points in its clinical applications. The points most frequently used are adjacent to the affected areas or the path of the related meridians. Pressing and digging on the acupuncture points is very similar to acupressure. Rubbing, stroking, pinching, kneading, and rolling are similar to massage, but manipulative methods go much deeper. Vibrating (or turning) is a special method to move joints and limbs passively by stretching the muscles, to stimulate the nerves around the joints, and to pull apart any adhesion of the joint capsule and ligaments.

Body work similar to Chinese manipulation has been used in SFAAHP, but acupressure is the chief method. This massage form is based on meridians and acupuncture points. Each massage lasts 30 minutes and usually is applied twice weekly. Patients enjoy these treatments and feel relaxed and refreshed after a session.

Chinese manipulation has specific methods for deficient conformations, using the tonifying massage to nourish blood, *yin*, and *qi*. The effects of tonification are similar to those of needling stimulation to the acupuncture points. Manipulation can work over a broader area, sometimes with even better results. Slow and gentle rubbing is the chief tonifying method for deficient patients. Rubbing around Cv 8 (*shenque*) can tonify spleen and stomach, rubbing the Gv 4 (*mingmen*) area can tonify kidney, and rubbing the Cv 17 (*tanzhong*) area can tonify lung. The tonifying rubbing should last at least 10 minutes and make the area warm and relaxed.

Some studies have been done to explain exactly how manipulation works. The most obvious sign of body ache is the spasm of the affected muscle, which can be shown by electromyography (EMG). Immediately after manipulation, the spasm waves on the EMG disappear, as does the pain caused by the spasm. Manipulation moves the joints and muscles to their extreme degree of extension, and this stretching can reflexively relax the muscles. Manipulation also can stimulate the nerves around the joints to increase the area's circulation, clearing the meridian pathways and regulating *qi* and blood. A similar mechanism will work for AIDS/ARC patients, giving a feeling of well-being.

Qi Gong (Breathing Exercises)

Qi Gong and AIDS

Qi gong is a hygienic breathing exercise. The meaning of the Chinese character "*qi*" is simultaneously the air we inhale and *yuan qi*, the vital energy of our bodies. The character "*gong*" means that it is a *gong fu* (alternatively spelled *kung fu*), mastery of a mental and physical achievement through systematic practice. This exercise is a method to regulate or condition vital energy in order to strengthen the body's ability to resist disease, to restore physiological functions, and to adapt to the external environment. It is an effective method of preventing disease and enhancing health.

Qi gong is also an exercise of the mind. It emphasizes the training of self-cognition and self-consciousness, using the mind to guide the movement of vital energy throughout the body. Through long-term training in *qi gong*, self-control and the mental ability to concentrate will be strengthened. This definitely will help with stability and calmness, allowing AIDS/ARC patients to be able to deal with their emotional and health problems in a more positive way.

Qi gong is an exercise of physical and mental relaxation. Mental relaxation is essential for relieving the stress from which AIDS/ARC patients suffer (Ann A. Cohen 1987). As fear, anxiety and uncertainty are endemic, *qi gong* is a very beneficial technique for relaxing the mind. *Ru jing*, or entering into mental quietness, is the basic requirement of *qi gong*.

Qi gong is a massage for the internal organs. With smooth, deep abdominal breathing, the diaphragm moves up and down regularly, effecting a gentle massage for all internal organs. During a *qi gong* exercise, this movement of the diaphragm may reach three to four times as far as it does in ordinary breathing; the narrow, deep, long, slow, steady, soft, and even breathing has a healing effect on the functioning of the lungs, heart, stomach, and intestines.

Qi Gong and General Relief from Disease

Traditional Chinese Medicine holds that an abundant supply of *yuan qi* is vital to maintain good health and prevent disease. Before the disease occurs, cultivating *yuan qi* can prevent it; after a disease's attack, restoring *yuan qi* can speed up recovery. *Qi gong* conditions and nourishes this vital energy to improve physical stamina and health.

The serenity (*ru jing*) of *qi gong* is due to the internal inhibition of the cortex of the brain. Under such protection, environmental stimuli can be cut off, over-stimulated nerve cells in the cortex can be rejuvenated, and the excitability of the cortex can be neutralized. On this subconscious level, the originally suppressed sensation of self/body enters the perception of the brain, and the body can concentrate on working for itself. This is especially effective for conditions closely related to one's nervous system and mental state.

Under *qi gong* conditions, the body reduces its oxygen consumption by 31%, with the metabolic rate reduced by 20%. This energy-saving effect can restore depleted energy reserves, and is good for treating heat-type diseases, as well as restoring the energy level of the physically weak (Shao et al 1988).

How to Practice *Qi Gong*

One cannot master *qi gong* overnight. A novice must practice it regularly and consistently. Begin with easy methods, and learn more complicated ones later. First, learn proper breathing, then learn *ru jing* to enter mental quietness.

Practice time should be short at the beginning, about 15 minutes, and gradually prolonged. One must set a proper schedule and select the method of *qi gong* appropriate for one's health, fitness, and mood. The time one plans for *qi gong* exercise should be free from interference. When there are too many mental distractions, the *qi gong* should be postponed.

Don't attempt to force mental quietness. Distractions happen frequently at the beginning. One should not try too earnestly to get rid of them, but let them go with the assurance that the mind will come back and be quiet.

There are various types of *qi gong*. For AIDS/ARC patients, or for physically weak persons, one basic type is recommended: *jing gong*, a static form of *qi gong* with no body movement involved. Static *qi gong* is a preliminary form, with which everyone should start. The next form can be a dynamic one, *dong gong*, involving body movement under the suggestion of the mind, or as suggested by an instructor.

Fang Song Gong (Relaxation Breathing Exercise)

Fang song gong is the gateway to *qi gong* and is relatively easy to practice. The breathing and relaxation techniques of *fang song gong* are the preliminary requirement for all types of *qi gong*.

Preparation

For physically weak persons, lying on the back is the position most often used. Place two hands gently on the knees or aside the body. Keep the eyes partially closed. Close the mouth naturally and let the upper and lower teeth gently touch each other. The tip of the tongue should lightly touch the roof of the mouth. Maintain this posture comfortably and effortlessly.

Be relaxed and natural. Allow both the body and mind to relax. Loosen the clothes and belt, and keep the posture at ease. Adjust the posture to be free from constraints. Relax the muscles, especially the muscles of the lower abdomen. Relax the mind, put a happy expression on your face, and be quiet and calm. Concentrate the attention at the *tan tien*, which is approximately three inches below your navel. Do not force yourself to concentrate, but be completely natural. If distractions do occur, return your thoughts to the same spot again.

Inhale - Quiet, Exhale - Relaxation

Now start to be quiet and to relax, beginning with the head. Just think: "I'm relaxing my head, relaxing from the depth of my head outward to the surface." This relaxation will cover one cycle of breathing. When you inhale, think, "Quiet." When you exhale, think, "Relax." Then go on to relax the neck, using similar thinking and the same breathing cycle. Repeat in this way, step by step, from the head, neck, shoulder, arm, hands, chest, abdomen, waist, hips, thigh, and legs, to the feet.

After relaxing the feet, use the same technique to relax the whole body several times, then let the entire body relax. Pay attention to certain areas of the body which feel sore or uncomfortable, thinking, "I'm relaxing this area." This period can last as long as is desirable.

Don't end the exercise suddenly. Rub the hands to make them warm, then rub the face with warm hands. Gently massage the eyes, nose, chest, abdomen, lower abdomen, and waist ("the gate of life"). Tap the ears, touch the teeth, then stretch both arms and legs.

The Effects of *Qi Gong*

Although there is almost no documented data on *qi gong*'s effects on AIDS/ARC, the *Qi Gong* Institute of the Traditional Chinese Medical Academy of Shanghai conducted a five-year investigation of the effectiveness of *qi gong* in cancer therapies (Rong Rong Zheng 1987). Depending on the patient's condition, the conjunctive therapies included chemotherapy, radiation therapy, surgery, and TCM. The test group consisted of 100 patients observed for periods of six months, one year, two years, and five years.

Qi gong exercises were begun as an adjunct to the other methods of treatment. As patients practiced *qi gong*, their general vitality and leukocyte levels were raised, enabling them to withstand the other treatments on a more frequent basis. Typically, the side effects from chemotherapy and radiation therapy diminished. When the patient's health increased beyond a certain threshold, called *shan gong* (entering the *qi gong* state), the other therapies were gradually reduced, while the *qi gong* was emphasized until only *qi gong* was used as therapy. The effects of *qi gong* were carefully observed and laboratory testing of the immunological status of each patient was performed frequently.

To assess the efficacy of *qi gong*, the Institute used a rehabilitation index compiled for malignant tumor symptomology and tested plasma levels of leukocytes, cAMP, and IgG, which are all immunological factors.

The mean rise on the rehabilitation index for the 100 cases was 23.6% in the first six months. The one-, two-, and five-year studies, conducted with smaller test groups, showed that general health continued to improve. A full 20% returned to full-time work for three to five years.

There are some similarities between AIDS pathogenic changes and the side effects of cancer therapies. *Qi gong* can nonspecifically strengthen the ability of cancer patients to tolerate the harmful effects of chemotherapy and radiotherapy on their immune systems. So why should it not be able to do the same for AIDS/ARC patients in their fight against the HIV's harmful effects on their immune systems?

7

Pharmacological Data

In previous chapters, many herbs have been mentioned for their effectiveness in treating AIDS, ARC, and HIV (+) patients. Other herbs exist which could also potentially be used because of their pharmacological properties. Although our limited clinical experience in treating AIDS/ARC with TCM precluded any previous reference to them, this chapter is intended to supply wider information about herbs which exhibit antiviral (especially anti-HIV), immuno-enhancing, immuno-regulating, anti-protozoan, anti-fungal, anti-cancer, or tonifying effects.

Basic pharmacological findings can help readers to understand these herbs in modern scientific terms and to use this information in the formulation of more effective herbal combinations.

Antiviral Chinese Herbs

Antiviral herbs are mostly *qing re jie du* (heat-clearing and toxin-eliminating) herbs used in Traditional Chinese Medicine for feverish infectious diseases (Dharmananda 1988; Hsu 1986; Yusheng Wang 1983; Wu 1982). Warm (febrile) diseases are identified by fever, chills, bitter taste in the mouth, dry throat, ruddy complexion, dry stool, and yellowish urine. TCM recognizes four sub-patterns: exterior, interior, excess, and deficiency of heat.

In AIDS/ARC patients, heat usually is interior and deficient in nature. Only at the onset of HIV infection do patients show influenza-like symptoms of exterior and excess heat.

Compared with Western antiviral drugs, these herbs have the advantage of a wider virus-suppressing spectrum with fewer side effects. Some of them even have immuno-regulating effects.

The most important research in direct inhibition of the growth of HIV by crude extracts of Chinese herbs in vitro has been done by Drs. Chang and Yeung (Chang 1988). This work is worth discussing in greater detail. Their results will be cited here and the pharmacology of these herbs which can inhibit HIV growth will be discussed in a later section of this chapter.

In their work, 27 medicinal herbs reputed in TCM to have anti-infective properties were extracted by boiling under reflux. The extracts were tested for inhibitory activity against the HIV in the H-9 cell line at a concentration non-toxic to growth of the H-9 cells. Using a significant reduction (3 standard deviations below the mean) in the percentage of cells positive for specific viral antigens in three successive assays, as indicative of activity against the virus, 11 of the 27 extracts were found to be active.

One of the extracts, *Viola yedoensis,* was studied in greater depth. At a subtoxic concentration, *V. yedoensis* completely halted the growth of the HIV in virtually all experiments. It did not, however, inactivate the HIV extracellularly, nor did it induce interferon or inhibit the growth of *herpes simplex*, polio

Table 7-1 Antiviral Chinese Herbs

Botanical Name	Chinese Name	Antiviral Effects	LD50
Viola yedoensis	*zi-hua-di-ding*	HIV	low toxicity****
Arctium lappa	*niu-bang-zi*	HIV	low toxicity****
Andrographis paniculata	*chuan-xin-lian*	HIV, ECHO11	13.4g/kg
Lithospermum erythrorhizon	*zi-cao*	HIV, jinke 68-1 flu, polio, hepatitis	1.3mg/kg**
Alternanthera philoxeroides	*kung-xin-lian-zi-cao*	HIV, flu, encephalitis B, retrovirus, rabies virus	455.5g/kg
Lonicera japonica	*jin-yin-hua*	HIV, flu (PR8), herpes, orphan	53g/kg (mice)
Coptis chinensis	*huang-lian*	HIV, flu, hepatitis B, Newcastle disease	24.3mg/kg*
Epimedium grandiflorum	*yin-yang-huo*	HIV, polio, ECHO 6,9, Cox-sackie A9, B4, B5	36g/kg
Woodwardia unigemmata	*guo-ji-jue-guan-zhong*	HIV, flu (PR8, jinke 68-1,57-4,NewA1, Lee, C1232,D), GlandIII, polio II, Coxsackie, *herpes simplex*, encephalitis	1.7g/kg (mice)
Prunella vulgaris	*xia-ku-cao*	HIV	low toxicity****

Senecio Scandens	*qian-li-guang*	HIV	302.6g/kg***
Hypericum japonicum	*di-er-cao*	HIV, hepatitis B	no obvious toxicity
Scutellaria baicalensis	*huang-qin*	HIV, flu (PR8, Asian A) *xiantai*, adenovirus 7, rhinovirus 17	3.081g/kg*
Baphicacanthis folium	*da-qing-ye*	flu, mumps, encephalitis B	no obvious toxicity
Baphicacanthis rhizoma et radix	*ban-lan-gen*	flu, hepatitis A,B, encephalitis B, herpes, mumps	no obvious toxicity
Bupleuri radix	*chai-hu*	flu, smallpox gland	4.7g/kg (mice)
Forsythiae fructus	*lian-jiao*	flu (Asian A), nose-17	29.37g/kg (mice)
Ledebouriellae radix (siler)	*fang-feng*	flu, Columbia SK	
Taraxaci herba	*pu-gong-ying*	ECHO11, herpes	156.3g/kg
Polygonum cuspidatum	*hu-zhang*	herpes, ECHO9, ECHO11 adenovirus, hepatitis B, flu, encephalitis B, Coxsackie A,B, polio II	1363mg/kg*

*LD50 is given in the doses of chemical essences of the herb.

**LD50 is given in the doses of alcohol extract, IV injection.

***LD50 is given dependent on the herb produced in China; in some countries this herb is very toxic (Geissman, 1964).

**** Toxicity will be explained later in the text.

or vesicular *stomatitis* viruses in human fibroblast culture. Chang and Yeung concluded that Chinese medicinal herbs appeared to be a rich source of potentially useful materials for the treatment of HIV infection.

There are 20 herbs listed in Table 7-1. The antiviral spectrum and toxicities of each herb are given. Thirteen of them have inhibitory effects on the HIV. From an allopathic view, it may not be proper to list these herbs until they have been tested against the HIV virus; however, from a TCM view, if certain herbs have been proven effective against a certain virus in clinical trials, the same mechanism may work against another virus in the human body. TCM holds that any herb or drug taken into the body must first affect the body's metabolism so that it can more effectively fight the pathogen. Although the concept of an antivirus is an allopathic approach, TCM's principle of treating febrile infectious diseases (*qing re jie du*, heat-clearing-and-toxin-eliminating) with herbal remedies can give this approach a new meaning.

The toxicity of these herbs is very low, so they can be used safely for a long period, even over a lifetime, by HIV-infected persons.

The 13 herbs which showed inhibitory effects on HIV in vitro may also contribute to the treatment of various complications of AIDS. On the following pages, each of these herbs will be discussed in greater detail, considering the properties traditionally attributed to them, their clinical applications, the formulas in which they typically appear, and the most recent pharmacological findings concerning them.

● *Viola yedoensis*

Other species sharing the Chinese name of this herb have not been tested in vitro for inhibitory effects on HIV:

Amblytropis multiflora, Corydalis bungeana, Gentiana loureirii, and *Polygala japonica* Houtt. When the herb is prescribed for its anti-HIV effect, only *V. yedoensis* should be used. This herb has a bitter taste, pungent flavor, and cold property. It has the action of removing toxic heat and relieving inflammation. Traditionally, it was used for carbuncles, deep-rooted furuncle, scrofula, and malignant lesions.

Its main active ingredients are violanthin, vitexin, saponaretin, orientin and isoorientin (Xuoshan Liu 1979; Pan 1988). Besides inhibiting the HIV, it has been found to inhibit the tuberculosis bacillus and many gram-positive and gram-negative bacteria. Drs. Chang and Yueng found that *Viola* is not a virus-killer; it does not inhibit HIV extracellularly. This finding points to the participation of the cell's mechanism in this inhibition and is consistent with TCM theory that the host is the primary force in the healing process. Its toxicity is very low; traditional TCM materia medica literature classified it as a "non-toxic" herb.

Clinically, it has been used for different infectious diseases like lymph node tuberculosis and especially for viral infections like mumps. The famous Three Flower Combination uses it as the main herb for treating mumps. The ingredients of this formula are viola 120g, lonicera 30g, chrysanthemum 30g, and licorice 9g (Dinshan Chen 1987). From this formula we can see that the dose for this herb can be as large as 120 grams per day. For an HIV infection, however, the herb will be taken for a very long period of time, so the dose should be lessened to avoid possible accumulative toxicity. This herb may be used to counter tuberculosis, a common complication in AIDS.

● *Arctium lappa*

This herb has a pungent flavor and cool property. Traditionally, it is used for dispersing wind-heat, clearing the throat, ventilating lung, promoting eruptions, removing swelling, and dissolving toxins. Clinically, it has been used as a treatment for cough, sore throat, unerupted erythema, swelling ulcer, and carbuncle.

Active ingredients are arctiun arctigenin, isoarctigenin, and arachidic acid. Besides inhibiting HIV, it also inhibits *Diplococcus pneumoniae, Staphylococcus aureus*, and dermatomyositis in vitro.

Typical formulas used for sore throat and sinusitis contain arctium 30g, *Schizonepeta* 30g, and licorice 15g (*Zhong Yao Da Zu Dian,* Dictionary of Chinese Medicinal Herbs, p. 430). It has a mild purgative effect. If the patient has diarrhea, it should be used with caution.

● *Andrographis paniculata*

A. paniculata has a bitter flavor and cold property. Since it has heat-dispelling and toxin-eliminating actions, it is used for infectious diseases such as tonsillitis, bronchitis, pneumonia, acute enteritis, red dysentery, urethritis, nephritis, pustular dermatitis, and purulent otitis media.

The active ingredients of this herb are andrographolide, neoandrographolide, paniculide A, B, C, 14-deoxy-11-oxoandrographolide, and 14-deoxy-11-dehydroandrographolide. It can inhibit *Diplococcus pneumonia* and some *Spirochaetaceae.* Clinical trials showed that its therapeutic effects for bacillary dysentery are stronger than those of the Western-prescribed antibiotic chloromycin. It has also been used against tuberculosis. Since gastritis, tuberculosis, and various infectious diseases are involved in AIDS, this herb can be used not only to inhibit HIV, but also treat and prevent other infections.

● *Lithospermum erythrorhizon*

This herb has a cold property and a sweet, salty flavor. It disperses swelling, removes toxins and heat, cools blood, smoothes the intestines, promotes defecation, and promotes rash eruption. Clinically, it has been used for the treatment of tumors, swelling, constipation, and various infectious diseases.

The active chemical ingredients are shikonin, deoshyshikonin, acetylshiconin, β, β-dimethylacrylshikonin, isobutylshikonin, b-hydroxyisovalerylshikonin, and teracrylshikonin. Besides its antiviral effects, it is anti-bacterial and can inhibit gram-positive and gram-negative bacteria and sporular dermatomycosis. Its anti-oncotic effects have resulted in its use in treating burns and dermatitis, the latter being a common complaint among AIDS sufferers. It is the chief ingredient of the famous exterior-use *Lithospermum* Ointment, which consists solely of this herb and *tang-kuei*. Its blood-activating effects can stimulate cardiac activity by promoting circulation. When used for measles and smallpox, it can promote the eruption of the rash and hence expel the toxins. In TCM pediatrics, it has been used for preventing and curing measles and small pox.

● *Lonicera japonica*

This herb has a sweet flavor and cold property. It can clear toxic heat and is used for fever, dermal eruption, carbuncle, and dysentery. It is a chief ingredient of *Yin-qiao-san* Formula, which is used for the common cold. It is also frequently used for viral infections such as mumps and influenza.

The active chemical ingredients of this herb are luteolin, lonicerin, and inositol. Besides antiviral effects, it has been found in vitro to inhibit *Shigella dysenteriae, Salmonella typhosa, Escherichia coli, Staphylococcus aureus, Streptococcus hemolyticus,* and *Hemophilus pertussis.* An inhibitory effect on the tuberculosis bacillus also has been reported.

This herb has also been proved effective against complications of AIDS, such as tuberculosis, diarrhea, and pneumonic infections. For HIV-infected patients, a gargle made from this herb and licorice can help to reduce the incidence of various infections.

● *Coptis chinensis*

This is one of the most important anti-infectious herbs of TCM. It has a bitter flavor and cold property. It dispels heat, alleviates dampness, purges fire, and removes toxins. Clinically, it has been used for fidgets due to extreme heat, sensation of fullness in the chest and abdomen, diarrhea, abdominal pain, tenesmus, hemoptysis, epistaxis, and oral ulceration.

The active chemical ingredients of this herb are ferulic acid and the alkaloids berberine, coptisine, palmatine, jateorrhizine, and worenine. Pharmacologically, it has shown inhibitory effects on intestinal bacteria, with the same efficacy as a sulfa drug. Its bitter taste has a stomachic effect and helps in digestion. It also stimulates the activities of the gastrointestinal tract and the secretion of gastric pancreatic and bile juices, as well as saliva. It is effective in treating diarrhea, combating fungal infestations and prolonging sleep. When treating AIDS patients, this herb can be also used against tuberculosis and *Candida.*

● *Prunella vulgaris*

This herb has a bitter, pungent flavor and cold property. According to TCM theory, it has the therapeutic actions of dispersing liver heat and dissolving accumulations. Clinically, it has been used for treating goiter, scrofula, conjunctivitis, carbuncle, wounds, ocular swelling and pain, photophobia, excessive tearing, and pinkish leukorrhea.

The active chemical ingredients are oleanolic acid, ursolic acid, rutin, hyperoside, caffeic acid, vitamins B_1, C, K, tannin, essential oils, alkaloid, resin, and water-soluble inorganic salts (68% potassium chloride). Pharmacologically, it has shown anti-bacterial effects which inhibit *Bacillus dysenteriae*, *Staphylococcus aureus*, *Pseudomonas aeruginosa*, and *Eberthella typhosa* in vitro. In vitro, the aqueous extract (1:4) was shown to inhibit some common pathogenic skin fungi to varying degrees. The pulmonary tuberculosis index and pulmonary lesions in mice with experimental tuberculosis were slightly reduced by daily feeding of the herbal powder following the infection. These pharmacological findings have been used for treatments of hypertension, tuberculosis of cervical lymph nodes, and acute icteric hepatitis. The later two complications are frequently seen in AIDS patients. Its pacific effects on liver fire can be used to calm emotional disturbances in HIV-infected patients.

● *Senecio scandens*

This herb has a bitter flavor and cold property. According to TCM theory, it eradicates heat, destroys intestinal parasites, and clears vision. Clinically, it has been used to treat acute inflammatory diseases, hyperemia of the eye, nebula, dysentery, jaundice, influenza, septicemia, carbuncle, lesions and pimples, moist fungal infections, and lead poisoning.

Its chief active ingredients are flavonxanthin, chrysanthemaxanthin, flavone, β-carotenoid, and alkaloids. Pharmacologically, its 50% aqueous decoction is a potent bactericide against *Shigella dysenteriae* and *Staphylococcus aureus*. In vitro it can effectively inhibit *Trichomonas vaginalis*. When used for AIDS patients, this herb functions both as an anti-HIV agent and as a treatment for bacteria- or protozoan-induced diarrhea. It is also a remedy for blurred vision.

● *Epimedium grandiflorum*

This herb has a pungent flavor and warm property. Most anti-infectious herbs are cold in nature; theoretically, these cold herbs should not be used in a disease like AIDS, which represents a severe deficiency condition (*xu zheng*), or at the very least, they must be used in low dosages. For this reason, there is controversy over treating AIDS with such herbs. *Epimedium grandiflorum*, however, is a rare exception which actually has a warm property, and, therefore, is recommended for use as one of the main ingredients of anti-HIV formulas.

According to TCM theory, it has the following therapeutic actions: supplementing kidney, strengthening *yang*, and dispelling wind-dampness. Clinically, it has been used for treating impotence, weakness in the loins and knees, and arthralgia due to wind, cold, and dampness. As we have observed, kidney deficiency is a major constitutional change in AIDS patients who tend to have a weak kidney pulse, low or absent sex drive, impotence, and weakness in the loins and knees.

Its active chemical ingredients are icariin, olivil, icariresinol (leaf and stem), Ω-methylicariin, magnoflorin and vitamin E (root). Pharmacologically, it has an aphrodisiac effect, mainly because it stimulates the secretion of semen, causing the filling up of the scrotum and thereby stimulating the sensory nerves, indirectly promoting sexual desire. It can dilate the peripheral blood vessels and inhibit the vasomotor center in the brain, so it has been used as a hypertensive drug. In small dosages it causes diuresis, while at high dosages it acts against diuresis. Its anti-infectious effects are not only antiviral, but also inhibit bacteria, such as *Staphylococcus albus, Staphylococcus aureus, Neisseria catarrhalis, Diplococcus pneumoniae,* and *Hemophilus influenzae.* At 1% concentration, the herb inhibits the growth of *Mycobacterium tuberculosis* in vitro. Its viral-inhibitory effects can be seen in Table 7-1. Besides its direct inhibitory effects, this herb has shown immuno-enhancing effects by increasing the phagocytic ability of cells in inflammatory exudates of mice. In our newly designed anti-HIV formulas, this herb has been used extensively.

● *Woodwardia gemmata*

One of a large family of antiviral herbs generally called *guan zhong, Woodwardia gemmata* is known as *guo-ji-ju* in traditional medical literature. It has a bitter and sweet flavor and warm property, the importance of which has been discussed above. According to TCM theory, it has the following therapeutic actions: supplementing liver and kidney, strengthening tendons and bones, and dispelling wind-dampness. Clinically, it has been used for treating waist, back and knee pain, foot and knee debility, enuresis, leukorrhea, urinary frequency in elderly men, and bleeding from all kinds of ulcers.

Its active chemical ingredients are woodwardinic acid, alkaloids, essential oils, and vitamin E. Since it is one of only two warm-propertied herbs which are anti-HIV, its liver- and kidney-tonifying effects, and its effects on body aches, make it particularly desirable.

● *Alternanthera philoxerodies*

A newly-discovered herb, *A. philoxerodies* serves as a good example of the clinical applications of these anti-HIV agents (Wu 1982). In the treatment of measles, a test group used a decoction of the herb and found that the course of both the disease and the fever were thereby shortened. The rashes of the test group appeared and disappeared faster than those of the control group. During the extreme stage of the disease, fevers in the former were lower, and there were fewer complications.

When this herb was used to treat encephalitis B, the cure rate was as high as 89.55%, especially if the herb was administered during the early stage of the disease. An army hospital in China has used it to treat severe encephalitis B. They used 100% concentration in the injectable solution of the herb, or 500% concentration in the oral solution. The mortality rate has decreased from 50%, without use of the herb, to 13% when using the herb.

This herb has also been used to treat epidemic hemalytic fever at the same army hospital. In a controlled clinical test of 188 cases, the test group consisted of 96 cases, with the control group using conventional drugs and steroids. Results showed that the overall mortality rate of the test group was 3.14% compared to 17.39% for the control group. In 81.82% of the cases, the disease was controlled by the herb, with the quantity of urine output much higher in the test group.

When used for viral hepatitis, symptoms were eased after two to three days of administration of the herb. After about 10 days, the jaundice disappeared, and within 7-60 days, the SGOT (serum glutamic oxaloacetic transaminase) and SGPT (serum glutamic pyruvic transaminase) figures returned to normal. The results for treatment of acute hepatitis with jaundice were also impressive: jaundice disappeared within 5-16 days, and the lab test figures returned to normal in an average of 23.7 days.

A. philoxerodies has also been used to treat epidemiologic hemalytic conjunctivitis. Eyedrops made from this herb were used in 72 cases, compared with 27 control cases using an eyedrop of 0.25% concentration *Guttae chloramphenicoli*. The average recovery time for the test group was 2.76 days, compared with 6.18 days for the control group.

The toxicity of this herb is very low; the LD50 in mice is 455.5g/kg. In clinical practice, using 100% concentration of the intravenous infusion with the dosage of 20-30g/kg for normal persons, there were no adverse effects on the heart, liver, kidneys, brain, blood pressure, or blood counts.

Although the antiviral effects have only been tested in vitro and it has been shown that few viruses were inhibited by this herb, its clinical trials found a much wider spectrum of viral diseases that could be treated by this herb. There may be certain unknown mechanisms involved in its therapeutic effects.

A strong point of the allopathic approach is to be specific; for example, AZT blocks the transcriptase of HIV. If we could disclose every drug's mechanism in this way, we could administer drugs in anticipation of that mechanism, and the HIV infection might be overcome much more easily. However, there is a great chasm between the present state of medicine and that point. Nevertheless, the specificity of drug mechanisms are no guarantee that toxicity and side effects won't hurt the human body. AZT badly damages blood-generating functions, a factor which has limited its usefulness in treating AIDS patients. The attempt to use an approach which is not so specific is, therefore, a reasonable step. The herbs discussed here may mobilize certain bodily functions instead of directly inhibiting the virus' reproduction or destroying the virus. This is a topic for more research.

In Drs. Chang and Yueng's research, the HIV-inhibitory effect of *Viola yedoensis* did not directly destroy the virus, or work extracellularly, though to inhibit HIV, the existence of H9 cells was a necessary condition. This also gave us a clue that certain cellular mechanisms must be involved in the inhibition of HIV. This phenomenon cannot be explained by the allopathic theory.

● *Scutellaria baicalensis*

S. baicalensis is bitter and cold in TCM pharmacology. It is credited for its dampness-heat-clearing, heat-purgative, detoxifying, and anti-inflammatory actions, and is known to prevent abnormal fetal movements. It is, therefore, useful against fever, cough (with thick sputum), pneumonia, hemoptysis, jaundice, hepatitis, dysentery, acute conjuctivitis, abnormal fetal movements, hypertension, carbuncle, and furuncle.

Its root contains five flavonoids: baicalein (scutellarein), baicalin (scutellarein-7-glucuronide), wogonin, wogonside (wogonin-7-glucuronide), and neobaicalein. The root contains β-sitosterol, benzoic acid, and an enzyme of *huangqin*. The stem and leaf contain scutellarin and baicalin.

Besides its antiviral effects, it has a wide anti-bacterial spectrum. Different degrees of anti-bacterial activity were exhibited, in vitro, by the *huangqin* decoction against *Staphylococcus aureus, Diplococcus pneumoniae, Streptococcus hemolyticus, Neisseria meningitidis, Shigella dysenteriae, Corynebacterium diphtheriae, Bacillus anthracis, Escherichia coli, Pseudomonas aeruginosa, Salmonella typhosa, Salmonella paratyphi, Proteus vulgaris*, and *Vibrio cholerae*. The decoction has shown a therapeutic effect on experimentally-induced tuberculosis in mice, but not in guinea pigs. The extract of *huangqin* was shown, in vitro, to be active against 10 kinds of skin fungi, including *Trichophyton violaceum* and *Microsporum audouini*, whereas the decoction was active against 9 kinds of skin fungi, including *T.violaceum* and *M.canis*.

Besides anti-microorganism effects, it has also showed anti-allergic, anti-inflammatory, sedative, anti-pyretic, hypotensive, diuretic, cholagogic, anti-cholera, spasmolytic, and detoxicant effects. Clinically, it has been used for treating chronic bronchitis, scarlet fever, and respiratory tract infections in children, as well as carriers of epidemic cerebrospinal meningitis, bacillary dysentery, leptospirosis, infectious hepatitis, acute biliary tract infections, and hypertension.

For treating AIDS, it is one of the chief ingredients of many heat-clearing and detoxification formulas of TCM, such as Coptis and Scute Combination and Minor Bupleurum Combination. Japanese researchers recently reported that, as the main ingredient of Minor Bupleurum Combination, *Scutellaria* had a strong inhibitory effect on the reverse transcriptase activities at concentrations less than 50 micrograms/ml, a dosage which is clinically attainable. At this concentration, the cellular DNA polymerases were not injured (Ono 1989).

● *Hypericum perforatum*

Hypericum is the Western herb St. John's wort. In TCM, it is called *di-er-cao*, or *tian-ji-huang*. Hypericin is its main active chemical ingredient. Herbal extracts chemically standardized for hypericin content have been sold over the counter as anti-depressants in Europe. In China, this herb has been used to treat hepatitis B.

Hypericin has also shown potent anti-retroviral activity in in-vivo tests with mice infected with two viral diseases. Furthermore, hypericin has been shown to inhibit HIV in vitro, apparently by a novel mechanism which blocks several different steps in HIV reproduction (Hebert 1989).

Immuno-Regulating Chinese Herbs

The material presented in this section is gleaned from two important books by Lu Heshen, professor of pharmacology at Guangzhou College of Traditional Chinese Medicine in Guangtong province, China. These texts have not been translated into English, but their titles may be translated as *Chinese Medicine and Immunity: Volume 1, Chinese Tonics* and *Volume 2, Blood-Regulating Herbs.*

TCM Tonics

Most immuno-enhancing and immuno-regulating Chinese herbs are TCM tonics, which evidence three main effects on immune functions: immuno-enhancement, selective immuno-suppression, and immuno-regulation. All of these properties are useful in treating AIDS/ARC patients (Geng 1988).

These herbs have been used for centuries as tonics in TCM, so it has been proven that their toxicity is very low, that they can be used safely, and that they can be used over an extended period.

The most extensively studied herb of this category is *Astragalus membranaceus* (*huangqi*), the most important *qi* tonic in TCM (Geng 1986; Lu 1982; Wagner 1985). It is the chief ingredient of a famous immuno-enhancing formula, Jade Screen Formula. The *fuzheng* formulas used for SFAAHP are the modifications of this formula and *huangqi* is the major component.

● *Affecting White Blood Cells (WBC)*

0.3 cc of 100% *huangqi* solution injected into mice subcutaneously for five days increased WBC counts (p). In clinical use, when *huangqi* was administered for chronic bronchitis, the rate of WBC phagocytosis increased.

● *Affecting the Reticular-Endothelium System*

Huangqi increases phagocytosis, thereby increasing the speed of clearing foreign particles. If combined with ganoderma, this effect can be strengthened. An interesting phenomenon is that this phagocytosis and the resulting clearing effect become more obvious after the reticular-endothelium system has been blocked (damaged) by carbon particles. This may explain why *huangqi* has better therapeutic effects on immunodeficient conditions. *Huangqi* and its combination (*Tangkuei* and Astragalus Combination) have been shown to increase the phagocytosis of macrophages of the spleen and abdominal cavity. In vitro, *huangqi* solution can dramatically increase the phagocytosis of *Streptococcus* by macrophages from the lungs of mice. Histochemical studies with electronic microscopy found that the polysaccharides of this herb are the active components responsible for this effect.

● *Affecting Interferon*

Huangqi can promote the interferon-producing ability of mice induced by the attack of the Newcastle disease virus ($p < 0.01$). After the attack of the Bimiti bunyavirus or NDV virus, the quantity of interferon in the lung serum shows dramatic increase, if *huangqi* is administered. In clinical trials, with patients susceptible to the common cold, the administration of *huangqi* increased the interferon-producing ability of the WBC induced by the virus ($p < 0.01$), the increase of this ability paralleling a decrease in the number and intensity of cold episodes. In vitro, 0.05-0.4% *huangqi* solution added to the spleen-cell culture of mice can induce the cells to produce γ-interferon, and *huangqi* can also increase the sensitivity of the cell to the interferon.

● *Affecting cAMP and cGMP*

Huangqi increases cAMP in human and mice blood plasma. Administration of *huangqi* or Jade Screen Formula can regulate the quantities of cAMP and cGMP in mice spleens. This effect is closely related to the antibody-producing cells of the spleen. The proper quantity of cAMP can reinforce the effects of interferon and the antibodies.

● *Affecting Production of Antibodies*

Healthy people were given 16 g raw *huangqi* for 20 days, and both serum IgM and IgE increased ($p < 0.05$). Those with deficiency symptoms were more greatly affected than those with symptoms of excess. Up to 40 days, IgG also increased. In a group of 83 chronic bronchitis patients, administration of *huangqi* solution for 20 days by injection resulted in increases of IgG, IgA, and IgM ($p < 0.01 - 0.001$). *Huangqi* solution can also increase sIgA in the sputum of these patients ($p < 0.001$). The sIgA level in sputum parallels the incidence of the disease.

Huangqi can promote the transformation of the lymphoblast. *Huangqi*, therefore, has extensive effects on the functioning of the immune system, and it can enhance and regulate the immuno-functions of the body. These effects can be used in the treatment of AIDS/ARC patients, for whom immuno-enhancement is a basic treatment. Scientific studies have tended to verify the immuno-enhancing or immuno-regulating effects of this herb (Geng 1986; Yingzhen Yang 1987).

I. Herbs Affecting Cell-Mediated Immunity

The immunodeficiency of AIDS/ARC patients is most evident in cell-mediated immuno-functions. The following herbs should be emphasized.

Increasing T-Cell Counts

Botanical Name	Common Name
Asparagus cochinchinensis	asparagus (root)
Atractylodes macrocephala	atractylodes, white (rhizome)
Coix lachryma-jobi	coix (seed)
Coriolus versicolor	coriolus (sclerotium)
Epimedium grandiflorum	epimedium (leaves)
Ganoderma lucidum	ganoderma (whole)
Lentinus edodes	lentinus (whole)
Ligustrum lucidum	ligustrum (fruit)
Panax ginseng	ginseng (root)
Phaseolus vulgaris	phaseolus, white (bean)
Polygonatum sibiricum	*huang-jing* (rhizome)

Promoting Lymphoblast Transformation

Botanical Name	Common Name
Angilica sinensis, acutiloba	*tang-kuei* (root)
Astragalus membranaceus	*huangqi* (root)
Atractylodes macrocephala	atractylodes, white (rhizome)
Codonopsis pilosula	codonopsis (root)
Coix lachryma-jobi	coix (seed)
Coriolus versicolor	coriolus (sclerotium)
Epimedium grandiflorum	epimedium (leaf)
Ganoderma lucidum	ganoderma (whole)
Gelatin equi asini	gelatin, equine
Ligustrum lucidum	ligustrum (fruit)
Panax ginseng	ginseng (root)
Phaseolus vulgaris	phaseolus, white (bean)
Polygonatum sibiricum	*huang-jing* (rhizome)
Polygonum multiflorum	*ho-shou-wu* (whole)

Polyporus umbellatus	polyporus (sclerotium)
Rehmannia glutinosa	rehmannia (root)
Schizandra chinensis	schizandra (fruit)

Increasing the Number of
White Blood Cells

Botanical Name	Common Name
Acanthopanax senticosus	ginseng, Siberian (root)
Astragalus membranaceus	*huangqi* (root)
Cinnamomum cassia	cinnamon (twigs)
Codonopsis pilosula	codonopsis (root)
Cornus officinalis	cornus (fruit)
Ganoderma lucidum	ganoderma (whole)
Gelatin Equi asini	gelatin, equine
Ligustrum lucidum	ligustrum (fruit)
Millettia dielsiana	millettia (stalk)
Panax ginseng	ginseng (root)
Phaseolus vulgaris	phaseolus, white (bean)
Placenta Homines sapientis	placenta (whole)
Psoralea corylifolia	psoralea (seed)

Promoting Phagocytosis of
Neutrophilic WBC

Botanical Name	Common Name
Astragalus membranaceus	*huangqi* (root)
Atractylodes macrocephala	atractylodes, white (rhizome)
Dioscorea opposita	dioscorea (root)
Glycyrrhiza uralensis	licorice (root)
Panax ginseng	ginseng (root)

Increasing the Number of Mononucleic Macrophages

Botanical Name	Common Name
Coriolus versicolor	coriolus (sclerotium)
Glycyrrhiza uralensis	licorice (root)
Lentinus edodes	lentinus (whole)

Promoting Phagocytosis of Mononucleic Macrophages

Botanical Name	Common Name
Acanthopanax senticosus	ginseng, Siberian (root)
Angilica sinensis, acutiloba	tang-kuei (root)
Astragalus membranaceus	huangqi (root)
Atractylodes macrocephala	atractylodes, white (rhizome)
Codonopsis pilosula	codonopsis (root)
Epimedium grandiflorum	epimedium (leaf)
Eucommia ulmoides	eucommia (bark)
Ganoderma lucidum	ganoderma (whole)
Lentinus edodes	lentinus (whole)
Panax ginseng	ginseng (root)
Polyporus umbellatus	polyporus (sclerotium)
Psoralea corylifolia	psoralea (seed)
Rehmannia glutinosa	rehmannia (root)

II. Herbs Affecting Non-Specific Humoral Immunities

Inducing the Production of Interferon

Botanical Name	Common Name
Astragalus membranaceus	astragalus (root)
Phaseolus vulgaris (PHA)	phaseolus, white (bean)

(Astragalus can also promote the production of interferon by viral stimulations.)

Anti-Complementary Activities

Botanical Name	Common Name
Cinnamon cassia	cinnamon (twigs)
Lentinus edodes	lentinus (whole)

(These herbs have triggering effects on the C3 complementary.)

III. Herbs Affecting Specific Humoral Immunities

Those Promoting Hypertrophy of Antigen-Combining Cells in Mice Spleens at the Early Stage of the Immuno-Reaction

Botanical Name	Common Name
Angilica sinensis	*tang-kuei* (root)
Astragalus membranaceus	astragalus (root)
Coix lachryma-jobi	coix (seed)
Cornus officinalis	cornus (fruit)

Those Promoting Hypertrophy of Antibody-Producing Cells

Botanical Name	Common Name
Asparagus cochinchinensis	asparagus (root)
Coix lachryma-jobi	coix (seed)
Coriolus versicolor	coriolus (sclerotium)
Epimedium grandiflorum	epimedium (leaves)
Ganoderma lucidum	ganoderma (whole)
Ligustrum lucidum	ligustrum (fruit)
Ophiopogon japonica	ophiopogon (root)
Polygonatum sibiricum	*huang-jing* (rhizome)
Polyporus umbellatus	polyporus (sclerotium)
Psoralea corylifolia	psoralea (seed)

Those Suppressing Hypertrophy of Antibody-Producing Cells

Botanical Name	Common Name
Glycyrrhiza uralensis	licorice (root)

Those Regulating Hypertrophy of Antibody-Producing Cells

Botanical Name	Common Name
Astragalus membranaceus	astragalus (root)

Those Increasing Antibody Production

Botanical Name	Common Name
Astragalus membranaceus	*huangqi* (root)
Coriolus versicolor	coriolus (sclerotium)
Epimedium grandiflorum	epimedium (leaves)
Lentinus edodes	lentinus (whole)
Panax ginseng	ginseng (root)
Placenta hominis sapientis	placenta, human
Polygonum multiflorum	*ho-shou-wu* (whole)
Rehmannia glutinosa	rehmannia (root)

Those Suppressing Antibody Production

Botanical Name	Common Name
Angelica sinensis	*tang-kuei* (root)
Glycyrrhiza uralensis	licorice (root)
Psoralea corylifolia	psoralea (seed)
Ziziphus jujuba	jujube (fruit)

IV. Those Herbs Affecting the Production of Different Types of Immunoglobulin (Ig)

Herbs Which Affect Immunoglobulin (Ig)

	Promotive	Suppressive
IgG	*Lentinus edodes* *Astragalus membranaceus*	*Psoralea corylifolia*
IgA (serum)	*Placenta hominis* *Rehmannia glutinosa*	*Psoralea corylifolia*
IgA (secretive)	*Astragalus membranaceus* *Ganoderma lucidum* *Polygoni multiflori* *Epimedium grandiflori*	
IgM	*Astragalus membranaceus* *Coriolus versicolor*	*Psoralea corylifolia*
IgE	*Astragalus membrananceus*	

Knowing which herbs can affect antibody production can also help with the formulation of herbal combinations for regulating the immune system.

Because of the disruption of the immune system, various allergic reactions can be seen in AIDS/ARC and HIV(+) patients, most notably hay fever and allergic sinusitis. The following are herbs which can be used for different types of allergic conditions.

I. Those Affecting Type-I Allergic Reactions

Those Suppressing the Secretion of Histamine

Botanical Name	Common Name
Ganoderma lucidum	ganoderma (sclerotium)

Those Providing Relief from Bronchial Spasms
Due to Histamine and Acetylecholine

Botanical Name	Common Name
Coriolus versicolor	coriolus (sclerotium)
Ganoderma lucidum	ganoderma (sclerotium)
Epimedium grandiflorum	epimedium (leaves)
Placenta hominis sapientis	placenta, human
Psoralea corylifolia	psoralea (seed)

Those Providing Relief of Gastrointestinal Smooth-Muscle
Spasms Caused by Histamine and Acetylecholine

Botanical Name	Common Name
Angelica sinensis	*tang-kuei* (root)
Cinnamomi cortex	cinnamon (twigs)
Cornus officinalis	cornus (fruit)
Glycyrrhiza uralensis	licorice (root)

Those Which Suppress Allergic Shock or Allergic Skin
Reactions Caused by Foreign Proteins

Botanical Name	Common Name
Glycyrrhiza uralensis	licorice (root)
Panax ginseng	ginseng (root)
Placenta hominis sapientis	placenta, human

II. Those Affecting Type-II Allergic Reactions (Cytolytic)

Those Preventing ABO Hemolysis

Botanical Name	Common Name
Glycyrrhiza uralensis	licorice (root)

Those Increasing the Number of Platelets

Botanical Name	Common Name
Glycyrrhiza uralensis	licorice (root)
Placenta hominis sapientis	placenta, human
Rehmannia glutinosa	rehmannia (root)

Those Increasing the Number of Red Blood Cells*

Botanical Name	Common Name
Acanthopanax senticosus	ginseng, Siberian (root)
Codonopsis pilosula	codonopsis (root)
Equi asini	equine gelatin
Panax ginseng	ginseng (root)

These herbs can also affect hemolysis.

III. Those Affecting Type-III Allergic Reactions

Botanical Name	Common Name
Astragalus membranaceus	astragalus (root)
Glycyrrhiza urlensis	licorice (root)
Rehmanniae radix	rehmannia (root)

IV. Those Affecting Type-IV Allergic Reaction (Delayed)

Botanical Name	Common Name
Angelica sinensis	*tang-kuei* (root)
Bombyx batryticatus	silkworm (whole)
Glycyrrhiza urlensis	licorice (root)

Clinical Applications

These herbs should be used according to the TCM differential diagnosis, as well as for specific immuno-deficient conditions. When they are used against infections, they may not directly suppress or kill the germs, but rather enhance the body's immuno-function and thus inhibit the infection.

When used as a treatment of cancer, immuno-enhancers alone are not very effective. If they are combined with radiotherapy or chemotherapy, the therapeutic effects can be enhanced while the side effects of chemotherapy or radiotherapy are reduced, an important consideration in the treatment of KS and malignant lymphoma patients.

Complications of AIDS/ARC Patients

Opportunistic Infections

Opportunistic infections ultimately develop in almost every AIDS patient. Most develop multiple infectious processes and die, either because there is no effective therapy available for the pathogen or because they no longer respond to conventional anti-microbial agents. Few AIDS patients die as a direct result of a tumor. In almost all cases, death is due to infectious complications. Thus, the quality and duration of patient survival is dependent on the ability to treat infections.

Because of the underlying immunodeficiency, patient response to treatment is poor. Once medication is stopped, the relapse rate is almost 100%, therefore, anti-infectious agents must be suitable for lifetime use. They must be very low in toxicity, with no severe side effects. It is difficult for chemically pure conventional drugs to meet these requirements, so herbs with anti-infectious properties can be very useful.

The clinical manifestations of opportunistic infections can be catalogued according to the pathogenic agents. The common infections are:

- protozoal infections (*Pneumocystis carinii, Toxoplasma gondii, amebae*, and *Cryptosporidium*)

- fungal infections (*Candida* species and *Cryptococcus neoformans*)

- bacterial infections [*Mycobacterium avium*-intracellular (MAI) and *Mycobacterium tuberculosis*]

- viral infections [Cytomegalovirus (CMV), *herpes simplex*, herpes zoster, and Epstein-Barr virus (EBV), hepatitis B]

Anti-Protozoal Herbs

Herb	Chinese Name	Protozoa	LD50
Allium sativum	*dasuan*	ameba, trichomonad	600mg/kg*
Artemisia annua	*qinghuo*	malaria	5105mg/kg*
Bupleurum chinense	*chaihu*	malaria	4700mg/kg
Coptis chinensis	*huanglien*	trichomonad, ameba	24.3mg/kg*
Dichroa febrifuga	*changshan*	malaria, ameba	7.79mg/kg*
Omphalia lapidescens	*leiwan*	trichomonad	insufficient data
Phellodendron amurense	*huangbo*	trichomonad	2.7g/kg
Pulsatilla chinensis	*baitouweng*	ameba, trichomonad	60g/kg

* The LD50 is given for the active principle of the herb.

TCM anti-protozoal herbs have been used in the People's Republic of China for treatment of amebic, malarial, and trichomonal infections. Their effects on AIDS-related protozoa have not been directly observed, but the same mechanism may be utilized in treating them. Clinical trials of the herbal treatment of diarrhea caused by *Cryptosporidium* have been encouraging (see Chapter 5).

Among these herbs, *Artemisia annua* (*qinghuo*) has been intensively investigated for its anti-malarial effects. This is an important herb in treating AIDS/ARC patients and we have used it frequently in SFAAHP. The herb has been used for many centuries in Traditional Chinese Medicine as a treatment for fever and malaria, specially for deficiency fever, which is common in AIDS/ARC patients. It is the chief herb in formulas for the anti-phlogistic treatment of MAI and tuberculosis, and is also used to compensate for the heat-producing properties of young deer horn. Its anti-malarial agents have been extracted from the leafy portions of the plant. The compound has been used successfully by several thousand malaria patients in China, including those with both chloroquine-sensitive and chloroquine-resistant strains of *Plasmodium falciparum* (Klayman 1985). The toxicity of this herb is extremely low, so it may be used safely.

Anti-Fungal Herbs

Anti-fungal herbs belong to the heat-clearing category of TCM herbs. Most fungal infections occur on the surface of the body on the skin or on mucous membranes. When the immune function of the patient has been damaged, the fungal infection can be disseminated to the internal organs. TCM considers surface fungal infections to be dampness-heat and internal organ fungal infections to be dampness-heat blended to and stagnated within the body. Because fungal infections in AIDS/ARC patients indicate asthenic heat, the herbs used to treat these infections should be mild and dampness-eliminating.

Anti-Fungal Herbs

	Chinese Name	Fungal Infection	LD50
Allium sativum	*dashuan*	*Candida, Cryptococcus*	600mg/kg
Coptis chinensis	*huanglien*	13 fungal skin infections of *Candida*	24.3mg/kg*
Houttuynia cordata	*yuxincao*	*Candida, Cryptococcus*	1.6g/kg
Phellodendron amurense	*huangbo*	fungal skin infections	2.7g/kg
Pseudolarix amabilis	*tujingpi*	*Candida*, fungal skin infections	insufficient data
Rosa cymosa	*yeqiangweigen*	*Candida*, deep fungal infections	insufficient data
Solidago decurrens	*yizhihuanghua*	fungal vaginitis, *Candida*, deep fungal infections	insufficient data

Coptis has been extensively used as an anti-*Candida* agent in TCM. It has been used both internally as a chief ingredient of anti-*Candida* formulas and externally as a single herb decoction to wash the affected areas. Its active anti-bacterial essences are berberine, coptisine, and ubrenine, which have been extensively studied for their anti-bacterial, anti-fungal, and antiviral effects. Having a wide anti-bacterial spectrum, *Coptis* can inhibit *Staphylococcus, Streptococcus lanceolatus, Bacillus dysenteriae,* and *B.anthracis*; it is a more potent agent against bacteria than penicillin. It can also inhibit *Bacillus pertussis, B.pestis, B.tuberculosis, B.typhi, B.proteus vulgaris,* and

B.diphtheriae. In addition, it also has been tested for anti-fungal activity and has proved very effective against various infections of the skin and mucosae. Its antiviral and anti-protozoal effects have also been applied in clinical therapies. Therapeutically, it not only directly inhibits germs, but enhances the natural immunity of the body. Experimental tests have also shown that *Coptis* can detoxify the endotoxin excreted by bacteria and suppress inflammation. In the HY-project, we used it as the chief ingredient of our anti-*Candida* formula.

Anti-Bacterial Herbs

Qing-re-jie-du (heat-clearing and toxin-eliminating) herbs possess anti-bacterial effects which have been investigated since the 1930s. Among them, the sub-category *qing-re-sao-she* (heat-clearing and dampness-eliminating) is the most effective in combating anti-bacterial infections. Most of their active essences have been extracted and their mechanisms are known (Hsu 1986; Yusheng Wang 1983; Wu 1982; Jinghuang Zhou 1986). Since bacterial infections in AIDS/ARC patients can vary greatly, we will list some herbs that have been extensively used in infectious diseases and some that can be used in specific bacterial infections with similar symptom patterns.

Herbs can be used as anti-tubercular agents as well. The traditional approach to treating tuberculosis in TCM is to nourish *yin* and lower asthenic fire. This is a constitutional treatment without direct application to the tuberculosis bacteria. Combining anti-tuberculosis herbs with conventional methods improves therapeutic results. Three herbs have been tested in both in-vitro and clinical trials.

Anti-Bacterial Herbs

Botanical Name	Chinese Name	Bacterial Infections	LD50
Allium sativum	*dasuan*	wide-spectrum bacteriostat, both Gram (+) and (-)	134.9g/kg
Berberis soulieana	*shankozhen*	wide-spectrum bacteriostat, both Gram (+) and (-)	3.1g/kg
Coptis chinensis	*huanglien*	wide-spectrum bacteriostat, both Gram (+) (-), and tuberculosis	24.3mg/kg
Forsythia suspensa	*lienqiao*	wide-spectrum bacteriostat, both Gram (+) and (-)	24.85g/kg
Gardenia jasminoides	*zhizi*	staphylococcus, diplococcus	31.79g/kg
Houttuynia cordata	*yuxingcao*	wide-spectrum bacteriostat, both Gram (+) and (-)	1.6g/kg*
Phellodendron amurense	*huangbo*	wide-spectrum bacteriostat, both Gram (+) and (-)	520mg/kg
Pulsatilla chinensis	*baitouweng*	wide-spectrum bacteriostat, both Gram (+) and (-)	60g/kg
Scutellaria baicalensis	*huangqin*	wide-spectrum bacteriostat, both Gram (+) and (-)	3.081g/kg
Senecio scandens	*qianliguang*	wide-spectrum bacteriostat, both Gram (+) and (-)	302.6g/kg
Taraxacum mongolicum	*pugongying*	wide-spectrum bacteriostat, both Gram (+) and (-)	156.3g/kg

* LD50 is given for the active essence of the herb.

Botanical Name	Chinese Name	Bacterial Infections	LD50
Humulus lupulus	*bijiuhua*	TB, Gram (-)	175mg/kg*
Humulus scandens	*liecao*	TB, Gram (-)	175mg/kg*
Lysionotus pauciflorus	*shidiaolan*	TB, Gram (-)	low toxicity

*LD50 is given for the extract of the herbs.

Allium sativum (garlic) is an important herb in treating infectious complications in AIDS/ARC patients. In the People's
Republic of China, it has been used as an injection or in a
concentrated extraction and is rarely used in formulas. Its active essences are allicin, allistatin, diallyl thiosulfonate, and
diallyl disulfide. The first three are responsible for its anti-bacterial effects, while the fourth is responsible for lowering
lipids in the blood. Its therapeutic effects are based on the following pharmacological effects:

- It can inhibit *Staphylococcus aureus, Streptococcus
  pneumoniae, B.typhi, B.paratyphi, B.dysenteriae, B.diph-
  theriae*, and *B.pestis.* (Purple-skinned garlic is more
  potent than white-skinned.) Garlic has also shown
  powerful inhibitive effects on *B.tuberculosis*, skin fungi
  and mucosae infections. It is effective against *Candida*
  and *Cryptococcus neoformans*, and can inhibit *amebae*
  and *Trichomonad.*

- Garlic has obvious immuno-enhancing effects. Experimental tests with mice showed that the administration of garlic can promote phagocytosis in mice. In
  human subjects, lymphocyte transformation rates
  dramatically increased with its administration.

- Allistatin has a suppressive effect on inflammation
  caused by formic aldehyde in rats.

● Garlic improves digestion and appetite.

● Experimental tests have shown that garlic extracts have suppressive effects on S180 sarcoma in mice, lymphosarcoma in rats, breast cancer in mice, and ascitic cancer and sarcoma in mice.

Since garlic has so many beneficial effects on a variety of infections and carcinomatic disorders, taking it regularly is an important measure for AIDS/ARC patients' daily hygiene.

Herbs for Cancer Treatment

The fact that HIV damages cell-mediated immunity may have oncogenic implications and the incidence of malignant tumors is to be expected in AIDS/ARC patients. Most frequently seen are Kaposi's sarcoma (KS) and primary lymphoma. KS is a disseminated vascular tumor, and primary lymphoma causes neurologic disorders and generalized lymphadenopathy. In conventional medicine, there is either no effective treatment for these cancers or the treatment exacerbates the underlying immunodeficiency.

TCM treatment for cancer has two basic approaches: *fuzheng* (immuno-enhancing) and "toxins to attack toxins" (using cytotoxic herbs to inhibit cancer-cell growth). Since these herbs are mostly toxic, they are used with other herbs which can compensate for their toxicity. These herbs belong to the categories of "soften the hard lumps and dispel the nodes." They have been tested in vitro and also have been extensively used in clinical treatment for many years. Some of their active essences have been chemically determined and investigated in vitro or in clinical trials.

Herbs With Anti-Cancer Effects

● *Cephalotaxus fortunei* (*shanjiensan*)

The active essences of this herb are harringtonine, homoharringtonine, deoxyharringtonine, and isoharringtonine. Its effects have been tested in mice for the inhibition of Walker carcinosarcoma 256 (W256), leukemia, sarcoma 180 (S180), and sarcoma encephaloid. In clinical trials, *shanjiensan* has been used to treat leukemia and malignant lymphoma. The effectiveness rate is 72.7% for leukemia and 60.8% for malignant lymphoma. Among these cases, about 20% had a complete remission. Clinically, the size of the lumps were usually reduced and the symptoms relieved. Its LD50 is 110mg/kg with its total alkaloid.

● *Crotalaria sessiliflora* (*nonjieli*)

The chief active essence is monocrotaline. Tests with mice showed that it can inhibit Ehrlich ascites (EA), S180, leukemia 615, adenocarcinoma, and W256. Clinical trials showed that it has some effect in treating dermal, cervical, penile, and rectal cancers. Its LD50 is 296mg/kg with its total alkaloid.

● *Curcuma zedoaria* (*ezhu*)

The chemical essences responsible for its anti-cancer effects are curcumol and curdione. Animal tests with mice showed that it can inhibit sarcoma. Tested with cancer-cell cultures in vitro, it can inhibit EA, leukemia, and vesical cancer U14. Clinically, it has been used for treating cervical, ovarian, and dermal cancers as well as malignant lymphoma. Remission rate for cervical cancer was 64.4%. Its LD50 is 16.75g/kg.

● *Sarcandra glabra* (*zhongjiefeng*)

The chemical responsible for its anti-cancer effects is flavone glucosides, which inhibits the growth of S180 cells and

W256 in vitro. Clinically, it has been used for treating stomach, pancreatic and esophagus cancers, as well as acute leukemia. Its LD50 is 24.75g/kg.

- *Robdosia rubescens (donglingcao)*

The chemicals responsible for its anti-cancer effects are rubescensine A and B. Cell culture tests showed anti-cancer activity against EA and liver cancer cells. Clinically, it has been used for treating esophagus cancer in its late stages. Its LD50 is 55.8mg/kg when treated with rubescensine.

- *Mylabris phalerata* Pallas (*banmao*)

Banmao is a small insect whose active ingredient, cantharidin, has been shown to inhibit the formation of liver cancer and S180 cells in vitro. It stimulates the bone marrow's blood-cell production and increases WBC counts. Clinically, it has been used for treatment of liver, esophagus, lung, and breast cancers. Relatively better therapeutic effects have been observed in the early stages of liver cancer. Its LD50 is 1.71 mg/kg.

- *Tripterygium wilfordii (leigongteng)*

The chemicals responsible for its anti-cancer activity are triptolide I, II, III, IV, V, and VI. Triptolide at 0.1mg/kg showed impressive life-prolonging effects in mice afflicted with L-1210 lymphoid leukemia. It has been tested on P388 leukemia and showed high inhibition at low concentrations. Its LD50 is 4.80g/kg with its raw herb decoction.

- *Catharanthus roseus (changchunhua)*

The active chemicals are vinceristine, vinblastine, and leurosine. Tests with mice showed that it can inhibit P-1534, L1210, Akr-leukemia, WM-256, IRC 741/1398 leukemia, S180, and EA. Clinically, it has been used for treating Hodgkin's disease, lymphoma, and acute lymphocytic leukemia. Its LD50 is 6.3mg/kg with its chemical essences.

● *Camptotheca acuminata* (*xishu*)

The active chemicals are camptothecine and hydr- oxycamptothecine. Animal tests showed that it can inhibit CA- 755, L-1210, and WM-256. Clinically, it has been used for leukemia and gastrointestinal carcinomas. Its LD50 is 68.4- 73.2mg/kg with its chemical essence.

● *Maytenus serrata* (*meidengmu*)

The active chemicals are maytansine and normaytansine. Animal tests showed that it can significantly inhibit P-388, S- 180, Lewis lung cancer, L-1210, and WM-256 at dosage levels in micrograms/kg. Clinically, it has been used for lung, breast, and ovarian cancers, as well as melanocarcinoma, lymphoma, and acute lymphocyte leukemia.

As a result of the extensive investigation of the herbs in this last group (Lien 1985; Wu 1983; Jinghuang Zhou 1986), there has been a tendency in clinical practice to administer their extracted chemical essences rather than the herbs in their traditionally processed forms. Nevertheless, this information is of considerable value in formulating herbal combinations for AIDS/ARC patients with carcinomatous complications.

Afterword

Never has a disease been identified so quickly or attracted so much attention by those in the medical profession and society as a whole as the AIDS epidemic. During the past year in which we have been collecting data and writing this book, both the epidemic and research aimed at combating it have advanced to new battlegrounds and new frontiers.

Thanks to conventional medical research, the life expectancy of AIDS patients has shown marked improvement. In 1982, only 30% survived 18 months following diagnosis. Today that percentage has more than doubled.

In the past year, there have been two international AIDS conferences, the scope of which are broadening to include a non-Western approach to the care and treatment of HIV-infected persons. Out of some 3,000 articles presented at the Fourth International Conference, held in Sweden in June of 1988, not one concerned Traditional Chinese Medicine, yet one year later, at the Fifth International Conference in Canada, three articles on the treatment of AIDS with TCM were accepted for presentation. Compared with 5,500 total, three is very small indeed, and as the second largest health-care system in the world, TCM surely should receive greater recognition for the benefits it can offer AIDS sufferers. Yet any progress, though it be slow and difficult, must always be welcomed.

During the course of our ongoing and intensive study of the treatment of AIDS with Chinese medicine, we have often asked ourselves the following questions: What outcome can we realistically expect from our research and the research of countless others? Can we totally eradicate the virus? If so, can we then rebuild the immune systems of those ravaged by the disease? We have gradually come to the belief that transforming AIDS into a manageable disease, i.e. a chronic viral infection such as viral hepatitis B or herpes, is probably the most we can expect.

According to known pathology, such a disease "metamorphosis" has three major stages: halting the reproduction of the virus; destroying infected cells, which act as "viral factories"; and rebuilding the immune system. Chinese medicine has shown progress in all three areas. The HIV-inhibitory properties of twelve herbs, for example, have been exhibited in in-vitro laboratory studies, the most recent discovery being scute by a team of Japanese researchers. Moreover, trichosanthin, the so-called Compound Q, as the active essence of *tian hua fen* (*Trichosanthes kirilowii*), appears to selectively destroy the infected T-cells and macrophages. Initial clinical treatments with this protein have shown very encouraging results. Combined with anti-HIV drugs such as AZT and DDI, we may yet be able to close the door on the HIV.

Halting the spread of the virus, however, is but one challenge facing us. The badly debilitated immune systems of hundreds of thousands, and perhaps millions, of people will also require major reconstruction and rejuvenation. Particularly in this realm, Chinese medicine can play a prominent role. The long history of TCM's treatment of the asthenic diseases *xu lao* and *lao zhai* provide a rich resource base from which to garner materials for the rebuilding of AIDS-impaired immune systems. Already several substances have been found to promote the production of T-cells and to regulate the immune functions, and through an integration of traditional knowledge and modern scientific research, it is now possible to develop even more effective immune enhancers.

The efficacious use of trichosanthin in the treatment of AIDS patients has provided a strong indicator of the beneficial results of such a synthesis of Eastern and Western medical practices and philosophies. Nearly 30 years of combining Chinese and Western medicine in China have established the groundwork for an integrated approach to diseases such as AIDS. In order to make the best use of this knowledge, physicians and patients alike must have open minds. For the patient's sake, the Western doctor must abandon preconceptions and biases, and embrace whatever can help the patient fight this battle and win. And for his own sake, the patient must take greater responsibility for his health and well-being than is generally afforded him by Western medicine.

Our personal research goals, and those of our colleagues, have gained greater clarity in recent years. We fully realize that to reach these goals much work must still be accomplished. AIDS is a very complicated syndrome, and many questions concerning it still lack even the most cursory of answers. We firmly believe that researchers such as ourselves would be negligent should we abandon our studies because our path is such a long and arduous one. Rather, we must not falter in our diligent search for safer and more effective treatments. Through close consultation and coordination, we are confident that traditional practitioners, conventional medical doctors, and our mutual AIDS, ARC, and HIV (+) patients can work together for the benefit of all.

1

The Diagnostic Standard of TCM Deficient Conformations

This standard was established by the Sub-Committee of Deficiency and Aging of the National Committee of Integrating Chinese and Western Medicine of China at their Guangzhou meeting in 1982. It was revised at their Zhengzhou meeting in May of 1986. The standard listed below is the revised version.

The diagnostic standard of deficient conformations involves the TCM concepts of *qi*, blood, *yin*, *yang*, heart, lung, spleen, stomach, liver, and kidney. For explanations of these terms, please refer to the glossary.

A. Deficiency of *qi*

The patient should have at least three of the following:

1. Low spirits, fatigue, and lack of energy

2. Shortness of breath, low voice, and unwillingness to talk

3. Spontaneous perspiration

4. Corpulent or jagged-looking tongue

5. Weak and powerless pulse (soft, small, and deep or superficial)

B. Deficiency of blood

The patient should at least have three of the following. If the patient has both these symptoms and those described in A, he or she has deficiency of both *qi* and blood.

1. Pale complexion

2. Dizziness upon standing

3. Pale lips and tongue

4. Fine pulse

C. Deficiency of *yin*

The patient should have at least three major symptoms and one minor symptom of the following. If the patient meets both these conditions and those described in A, the patient has deficiency of both *qi* and *yin*.

1. Major symptoms

    a. hot feeling in palms, soles, and chest

    b. dry throat and thirst

    c. red tongue with little or no fur

    d. fine and fast pulse

2. Minor symptoms

    a. "flushing up" in afternoons

    b. dry stools, constipation, and small quantities of dark-colored urine

    c. night sweats

D. Deficiency of *yang*

The patient should have at least three of the following major symptoms (the first is a must) and one of the following minor symptoms. If the patient meets these conditions as well as those of described in C, he/she has a deficiency of both *yin* and *yang*.

   1. Major symptoms

      a. chills in entire body, certain parts of the body, or in the extremities

      b. edema of face or feet

      c. pale and corpulent tongue with a moist coating

      d. submerged, slow, and indistinct pulse

   2. Minor symptoms

      a. frequent urination during the night

      b. loose stools and large quantities of colorless urine

E. Deficiency of heart

The patient should have at least two of the following, and the first item is a must. This deficiency usually appears along with *qi*, blood, *yin*, or *yang* deficiencies. As such, the corresponding conformations are heart *qi* deficiency, heart blood deficiency, heart *yin* deficiency, or heart *yang* deficiency.

   1. Palpitation and a compressed feeling in the chest

   2. Insomnia or dreaminess

   3. Memory loss

   4. Irregular or regularly-occurring intermittent pulse or fine and weak pulse

F. Deficiency of lung

The patient should have at least two of the following. Lung deficiency usually exists with *qi* or *yin* deficiencies.

   1. Persistent cough with white phlegm

   2. Shortness of breath

   3. Susceptibility to colds

G. Deficiency of spleen

The patient should have at least three of the following. Spleen deficiency usually exists with *qi*, *yin*, or *yang* deficiencies.

1. Loose stools or diarrhea
2. Stomach distension and flatulence after meals, relieved by pressing the stomach
3. Dim and yellowish complexion
4. Poor appetite
5. Weight loss; thin, with no energy

H. Deficiency of stomach

The patient should have at least two of the following. Stomach deficiency usually exists with *qi*, *yin* or *yang* deficiencies.

1. Stomachache, relieved after eating
2. Abdominal pain, relieved by pressing the abdomen
3. Poor or excessive appetite
4. Indigestion

I. Deficiency of liver

The patient should have at least three of the following. Liver deficiency usually exists with blood or *yin* deficiencies.

1. Dizziness and blurred vision (arcus senilis)
2. Numbness of limbs
3. Anxious, irritable, irascible and easy to anger, or depressed and sighing heavily in despair
4. Dry eyes

J. Deficiency of kidney

The patient should have at least three of the following. Kidney deficiency usually exists with *qi*, *yin*, or *yang* deficiencies.

1. Pain and numbness in back and lower back (discounting injuries)

2. Numbness in legs and knee joints, and pain in heels

3. Deafness or tinnitus

4. Hair loss and loose teeth

5. Declining amounts of urination or urinary incontinence

6. Impotence, infertility, or sterility

2

Criteria Established by the Center for Disease Control for the Diagnosis of AIDS and ARC

I. AIDS – Surveillance Definition of the Center for Disease Control

The occurrence of any of the below-listed diseases that is at least moderately predictive of a defect in cell-mediated immunity, occurring in a person with no known cause for diminished resistance to that disease

A. Kaposi's sarcoma (in patients less than 60 years of age)

B. Primary lymphoma of the central nervous system

C. *Pneumocystis carinii* pneumonia

D. Unusually extensive mucocutaneous *herpes simplex* of longer than 5 weeks' duration

E. *Cryptosporidium enterocolitis* of longer than 4 weeks' duration

F. Esophagitis due to *Candida albicans*, cytomegalovirus, or *herpes simplex* virus

G. Progressive multifocal leukoencephalopathy

H. Pneumonia, meningitis, or encephalitis due to one or
more of the following

   1. *Aspergillus*

   2. *Candida albicans*

   3. *Cryptococcus neoformans*

   4. Cytomegalovirus

   5. *Nocardia*

   6. *Strongyloides*

   7. *Toxoplasma gondii*

   8. *Zygomycosis*

   9. Atypical *Mycobacterium* species (excluding *tuberculosis* and *lepra*)

II. Pediatric AIDS – Provisional Surveillance Definition of the Center for Disease Control

Same as for AIDS in adults (given above), with the following provisions

A. Congenitial infections which must be excluded

   1. *Toxoplasma gondii* in patients less
than 1 month old

   2. *Herpes simplex* virus in patients less
than 1 month old

   3. Cytomegalovirus in patients less than 6 months old

B. Specific conditions which must be excluded

   1. Primary immunodeficiency diseases

     a. Severe combined immunodeficiency

     b. Di George's syndrome

     c. Wiskott-Aldrich syndrome

     d. Ataxia-telangiectasia

     e. Graft-versus-host reaction

     f. Neutropenia

  g. Neutrophil function abnormality

  h. Agammaglobulinemia

  i. Hypogammaglobulinemia with elevated IgM

 2. Secondary immunodeficiency associated with immunosuppressive therapy, lymphoreticular malignancy or starvation

III. Conditions Prompting an AIDS-Related Complex (ARC) Diagnosis (Must Meet the Conditions of A, B and C Below)

A. Any two of the following clinical features

 1. History of fever greater than 100° F and persisting three months or longer

 2. Weight loss in excess of 10%, or greater than 15 pounds

 3. Lymphadenopathy of at least 3 months' duration

 4. Diarrhea persisting 3 months or longer

 5. Night sweats

 6. Fatigue

B. Any two of the following laboratory abnormalities

 1. Helper T-cells less than 400/mm

 2. Helper:suppressor ratio less than 1.0

 3. Leukopenia (WBC less than 2,000)

 4. Thrombocytopenia (platelets less than 100,000)

 5. Anemia (HCT less than 35)

 6. Elevated serum globulins

 7. Depressed blastogenesis (phytohemagglutinin)

 8. Anergy to skin tests

C. One of the following test results

 1. positive HIV culture

 2. positive HIV antibody

Formulas

Aconite, Ginseng, and Ginger Combination
fu zhi li zhong tang
  ginseng, ginger, licorice, atractylodes, aconite

Agastache Formula
huo xiang zheng qi san
  agastache, atractylodes, pinellia, hoelen, magnolia
  bark, citrus, platycodon, angelica, perilla, areca,
  jujube, ginger, licorice

Anemone Combination
bai tou won tang
  anemone, coptis, fraxinus, phellodendron

Astragalus and Tortoise Shell Formula
huang qi bie jia san
  ginseng, cinnamon bark, pinellia, anemarrhena,
  peony (red), astragalus, licorice, tortoise shell, *chin-
  chiu*, hoelen, lycium root, rehmannia, bupleurum,
  asparagus, morus bark, platycodon, aster

Astragalus and *Zizyphus* Combination
yang xin tang
> astragalus, *tang-kuei*, biota, polygala, *fushen*, hoelen, pinellia, cinnamon, licorice, cnidium, ginseng, schizandra, *Zizyphus*

Astragalus Combination
huangqi jiang zhong tang
> peony, jujube, malt, cinnamon, licorice, ginger (fresh), astragalus

Astragalus Formula
huang qi san
> astragalus, peony (red), capillaris, gypsum, ophiopogon, licorice, soja

Atractylodes and Citrus Formula
bai zhu gao
> atractylodes (white), citrus, ginseng

Baked Licorice Combination
zhi gan cao tang
> baked licorice, ginger (fresh), linum, jujube, ginseng, ophiopogon, gelatin, rehmannia, cinnamon

Bupleurum and Cypress Combination
chia hu shu gan tang
> bupleurum, citrus fruit, peony (white), cypress, curcumae, malia fruit, citrus rind, immature citrus fruit, licorice

Capillaris Combination
yin chen hao tang
> capillaris, gardenia, rhubarb

Chin-chiu and Rehmannia Combination
qing gu san
> bupleurum, dried rehmannia, ginseng, siler, processed rehmannia, *chin-chiu*, mentha, hoelen, picrorhiza

Chin-chiu and Tortoise Shell Formula
qin gu bie jia san
> *chin-chiu*, *ching-hao*, mume, anemarrhena, *tang-kuei*, tortoise shell, bupleurum, lycium bark, ginger

Cinnamon and Astragalus Combination
guizhi jia huang qi tang
> cinnamon, peony, jujube, ginger (fresh), licorice

Cinnamon and Dragon Bone Combination
guizhi jialong gu mu li tang
> cinnamon, peony jujube, ginger (fresh), oyster shell, licorice, dragon bone

Cinnamon and Ginseng Combination
guizhi ren shen tang
> cinnamon, ginseng, licorice, atractylodes, white ginger (fresh)

Citrus and Pinellia Combination
fen xin qi yin
> citrus, cinnamon, peony, akebia, pinellia, areca, hoelen, *chianghuo*, morus, juncus, perilla, jujube, blue citrus peel, licorice, ginger

Clearing Heat and Nourishing *Yin* Formula
qing re yang yin san
> scrophularia, ophiopogon, rehmannia, *Adenophorae stricta, Sophorae subprostrata*, gardenia, coptis, astragalus, *Juncus*

Coptis and Scute Combination

huang liang jie du tang
    acute, coptis, gardenia, phellodendron

Dioscorea and Jujube Formula

shu-yu-wan
    dioscorea, ophiopogon, *tang-kuei*, apricot seed, cin-
    namon, bupleurum, yeast, platycodon, rehmannia,
    hoelen, licorice, bean sprouts, gelatin, dried ginger,
    ginseng, ampelopsis, cnidium, siler, peony, jujube,
    atractylodes

Forsythia and Laminaria Combination

san zhong kui jian tang
    tang-kuei, peony, bupleurum, scute, coptis, forsythia,
    phellodendron, platycodon, *Gentiana*, anemarrhena,
    pueraria, *Scirpus*, zedoaria, laminaria, seaweed,
    cimicifuge, ginger, licorice, *Trichosanthes*

Forsythia and Rhubarb Formula

liang ge san
    forsythia, rhubarb, scute, mirabilitum, licorice,
    gardenia, bamboo leaves, mentha

Four Major Herb Combination

si jun zi tang
    ginseng, atractylodes, hoelen, licorice

Gentiana Combination

long danxie gantang
    gentiana, alisma, akebia, *Plantago*, *tang-kuei*,
    rehmannia, gardenia, scute, licorice

Ginseng and Aconite Combination

shen fu tang
    ginseng, aconite, ginger, jujube

Ginseng and Astragalus Combination
bu zhong yi qi tang
> ginseng, licorice, atractylodes (white), citrus, *tang-kuei*, cimicifuga, bupleurum, ginger (fresh), jujube

Ginseng and Astragalus Formula
shen qi gao
> ginseng, astragalus

Ginseng and Atractylodes Formula
shenlingbai zhusan
> ginseng, dolichos, atractylodes (white), hoelen, dioscorea, lotus seed, coix, cardamon, platycodon, licorice

Ginseng and Dioscorea Formula
zhi-sheng-jian-pi-wan
> dioscorea, atractylodes (white), ginseng, hoelen, lotus seed, citrus, malt, *shen-chu*, coix, euryale, *Crataegus, Dolichos*, cardamon

Ginseng and Ginger Combination
ren shen tang
> ginseng, ginger, licorice, atractylodes

Ginseng and Gypsum Combination
bai hu jia ren shen tang
> gypsum, anemarrhena, *Oryza*, licorice, ginseng

Ginseng and *Tang-kuei* Ten Combination
shi quanda butang
> ginseng, atractylodes (white), peony, hoelen, rehmannia, *tang-kuei*, cnidium, cinnamon, licorice

Ginseng and *Zizyphus* Formula
tian wangbu xindan

rehmannia, ginseng, schrophularia, salvia, hoelen, platycodon, polygala, biota, asparagus, ophiopogon, *tang-kuei*, schizandra, acorus, cinnabar, *Zizyphus*, coptis

Ginseng Combination
ren shen yang rong tang

ginseng, *tang-kuei*, peony, rehmannia, atractylodes, hoelen, cinnamon, astragalus, citrus, polygala, schizandra, licorice

Ginseng Nutritive Combination
ren shen yang rong tang

ginseng, *tang-kuei*, peony, rehmannia, atractylodes, hoelen, cinnamon, astragalus, citrus, polygala, schizandra, licorice

Great Universal *Yin* Formula
da bu yin wan

phellodendron, anemarrhena, rehmannia, tortoise shell

HY-1
fuzheng - I

bupleurum, scute, pinellia, ginseng, jujube, licorice, ginger, astragalus, siler

HY-2
fuzheng - II

astragalus, siler, ginseng, *Polygonatum* root, epimedium, rehmannia

HY-3
quxie - I

isatis leaf, bupleurum, *Lithospermum*, licorice, citrus

HY-4
quxie - II
  isatis root, gardenia, *Blechnum*, licorice, citrus

HY-5
kang-ai - I
  tang-kuei, peony, cnidium, rhubarb, licorice, oyster,
  shell, *Cimicifuga*, astragalus, lonicera, *Lithospermum*

HY-6
he-jie - I
  bupleurum, scute, pinellia, jujube, ginseng,
  licorice, ginger

HY-7
qing-fei-re - I
  scute, platycodon, morus, apricot seed, gardenia,
  asparagus, fritillaria, citrus, jujube, bamboo, hoelen,
  ginger, *tang-kuei*, ophiopogon, licorice, schizandra

HY-8
qing-re - I
  ma-huang, apricot seed, licorice, gypsum

HY-9
zhi-xie - I
  pueraria, coptis, scute, licorice

HY-10
jian-pi - I
  ginseng, atractylodes, hoelen, citrus, licorice, pinellia
  Saussurea, cardamon

HY-11
kang-zhen-jun - I
  ginseng, licorice, ginger, atractylodes, coptis,
  gentiana

HY-12
huo-xue - I
tang-kuei, rehmannia, peony, cnidium, coptis, scute, phellodendron, gardenia

HY-13
kang-mei - I
akebia, cnidium, hoelen, licorice, lonicera, rhubarb, *Smilax*

HY-14
kang-gan-yan - I
capillaris, gardenia, rhubarb

HY-15
kang-gan-yan - II
capillaris, cinnamon, *Polyporus*, hoelen, atractylodes, alisma

HY-16
qing-xu-re - I
anemarrhena, phellodendron, hoelen, *Cornus*, dioscorea, alisma, moutan, rehmannia

HY-17
he-jie - II
tang-kuei, peony, gardenia, ginger, atractylodes, hoelen, mentha, bupleurum, licorice, moutan

HY-18
qing-xu-re - II
chin-chiu, qing-huo, mume, ginger, anemarrhena, *tang-kuei*, bupleurum, tortoise shell, lycium bark

HY-19
kang-ai - II

   tang-kuei, peony, bupleurum, scute, coptis, phellodendron, platycodon, anemarrhena, forsythia, gentiana, ginger, zedoaria, *Pueraria, Scirpus, Cimicifuga*, licorice, *Trichosanthes* root, laminaria, seaweed

HY-20
jian-pi - II

   ginseng, ginger, licorice, aconite, atractylodes

HY-21
chu-shi-re - I

   Gentiana, alisma, akebia, *Plantago*, scute, *tang-kuei*, rehmannia, gardenia, licorice

HY-22
fuzheng and quxie - I

   astragalus, siler, ginseng, salvia, isatis leaf and root, rehmannia, deer horn, *tang-kuei*, licorice, *Smilax, Cuscuta*, millettia

HY-23
bu-xue - I

   rehmannia, dendrobium, lycium fruit, *Ligustrum, Curculigo, epimedium, Morinda*

HY-24
huo-xue - II

   tang-kuei, peony, rehmannia, *Persica*, cnidium, carthamus

HY-25
zhi-xie - III

   mume, asarum, aconite, cinnamon, *tang-kuei*, phellodendron, ginseng, coptis, zanthoxylum, ginger

HY-26

zhi-xie - IV

anemone, coptis, *Fraxinus*, phellodendron

HY-27

zhi-xie - V

anemone, coptis, *Fraxinus*, phellodendron, brucea, dichroa root, *Sanguisorba*, *Terminalia*

HY-28

bu-xue - II

antler (young), salvia, *qing-hao*

HY-30

fuzheng and *quxie* - II

viola, lonicera, epimedium, licorice, astragalus, *Ligustrum*, *Ganoderma*

HY-31

fuzheng and *quxie* - III

viola, epimedium, coptis, prunella, licorice, astragalus, cassia seed

HY-32

jian-pi - III

ginseng, *Colichos*, atractylodes, hoelen, dioscorea, lotus seed, coix, cardamon, platycodon, licorice

HY-33

qing-xu-re - III

gypsum, anemarrhena, *Oryza*, licorice, ginseng

HY-34

zhi-dao-han - I

tang-kuei, rehmannia, astragalus, coptis, scute, phellodendron

HY-35
zhi-dao-han - II
  astragalus, atractylodes (white), siler, ginger

HY-36
bu-yi - I
  astragalus, ginseng, licorice, atractylodes, citrus, *tang-kuei*, *Cimicifuga*, ginger, bupleurum, jujube

HY-37
bu-yi - II
  ginseng, astragalus, atractylodes, peony, hoelen, rehmannia, *tang-kuei*, cnidium, cinnamon, licorice

HY-38
qu-tong - I
  salvia, peony (red), moutan, *Persica, chin-chiu,* cinnamon twigs, *tu-huo*, corydalis

HY-39
kang-lao - I
  prunella, *Ulva*, oyster shell, scrophularia

Kao-ben and Cnidium Combination
bao zheng tang
  kao-ben, cnidium, licorice, atractylodes

Kidney-and-Spleen-Nourishing Pill
zhi sheng jian pi wan
  dioscorea, atractylodes, ginseng, hoelen, lotus seed, citrus, malt, coix, cardamon, *Dolichos, Crataegus,* euryale, *shen-chu*

Lily Combination
bai hegu jintang
  lily, peony, *tang-kuei*, fritillaria, licorice, rehmannia, ophiopogon, figwort, platycodon

Lithospermum and Oyster Shell Combination
zi gen muli tang

> *tang-kuei*, peony, cnidium, oyster shell, rhubarb, cimicifuge, astragalus, licorice, lonicera, *Lithospermum*

Liver-Tonifying Combination
bu gan tang

> *Cornus*, licorice, cinnamon, hoelen, siler, aconite, *Persica*, asarum, *Biota*

Lonicera and Forsythia Formula
yin qiaosan

> lonicera, forsythia, platycodon, *Arctium*, mentha, licorice, bamboo leaves, *Schizonepeta, Soja, Phragmites*

Lung-Tranquilizing Combination
nin fei tang

> scute, fritillaria, anemarrhena, *Trichosanthes* root, *Asparagus*, apricot seed, morus bark, *Glehnia, Eriobotrya*

Machixian Jiedu Decoction

> *Portulaca oleracea*, isatis, *Lithospermum, Patrinia*, coptis, *Zizyphus*, oyster shell

Magnolia and Hoelen Combination
wei ling tang

> atractylodes (white), magnolia bark, citrus, jujube, ginger (fresh), licorice, hoelen, *Polyporus*, alisma, cinnamon

Major Five Organs Tonifying Formula
da wu bu wan

ginseng, rehmannia, ophiopogon, lycium fruit, lycium root, *fu-shen*, Asparagus, Alpinia fruit, *Acorus, Polygala*

Major *Yuan Qi* Tonifying Formula
da bu yuan jian

dioscorea, eucommia, rehmannia, *tang-kuei, Lycium* fruit, baked licorice, *Cornus*

Minor Bupleurum Combination
xiao chai hu tang

bupleurum, pinellia, ginger, scute, ginseng, jujube, licorice

Minor Cinnamon and Peony Combination
xiaojian zhongtang

cinnamon, ginger (fresh), peony, jujube, licorice, malt

Pacific Formula
tai bing wan

Asparagus, ophiopogon, anemarrhena, apricot seed, *tang-kuei*, raw rehmannia, coptis, gelatin, mentha, fritillaria, platycodon, tussilago, bulrush, musk

Platycodon and Fritillaria Combination
qing fei tang

scute, platycodon, morus, apricot seed, gardenia, *Asparagus*, fritillaria, citrus, jujube, bamboo, hoelen, ginger, *tang-kuei*, ophiopogon, licorice, schizandra

Pueraria, Coptis, and Scute Combination
shen ling bai zhu san

ginseng, *Dolichos*, atractylodes, hoelen, dioscorea, lotus seed, coix, cardamon, platycodon, licorice

Rehmannia and Akebia Formula
dao chi san
rehmannia, akebia, *Lophatherum*, licorice

Rehmannia Eight Formula
ba weide huangwan
rehmannia, cinnamon, aconite, hoelen, dioscorea, alisma, moutan, *Cornus*

Rehmannia Six Formula
liu wei de huang wan

Rhubarb and *Eupolyphaga* Formula
da-huang-zhe-zhung-wan
steamed rhubarb, dried rehmannia, scute, dried lacquer, licorice, leech, peony, *Tabanus, Persica, Holotrichia,* apricot seed, *Eupolyphaga*

***Saussurea* and Cardamon Combination**
xiang shaliu jun zitang
ginseng, atractylodes (white), hoelen, licorice, pinellia, citrus *Saussurea*, cardamon

***Tang-kuei* and Astragalus Combination**
dang gui bu xie tang
astragalus, *tang-kuei*

***Tang-kuei* and Bupleurum Formula**
xiao yao san
tang-kuei, peony, mentha, bupleurum, ginger, licorice, hoelen, atractylodes

***Tang-kuei* Four Combination**
si wutang, tang-kuei, peony, cnidium, rehmannia

Three Flower Combination
san hua tang
> lonicera, viola, chrysanthemum, licorice

Tortoise Shell and Rehmannia Combination
bie jia ti huang tang
> bupleurum, *tang-kuei*, ophiopogon, tortoise shell, atractylodes, rehmannia, hoelen, *chin-chiu*, ginseng, cinnamon bark, baked licorice, ginger, dendrobium

Yang-Lifting and *Lao*-Nourishing Combination
cheng yang li lao tang
> astragalus, ginseng, cinnamon Bark, *tang-kuei*, citrus, atractylodes (white), licorice, schizandra, ginger, jujube

Yang-Lifting and Stomach-Nourishing Combination
shen yang yi wei tang
> astragalus, pinellia, ginseng, baked licorice, peony (white), siler, citrus, hoelen, alisma, bupleurum, atractylodes, coptis, *tu-huo, chiang-huo*

Yin-Lifting and *Lao*-Nourishing Combination
cheng yin li lao tang
> moutan, *tang-kuei*, ophiopogon, citrus, baked licorice, coix, lotus seed, peony (white), schizandra, ginseng, rehmannia, jujube

Zizyphus Combination
suan chao ren tang
> *Zizyphus*, hoelen, cnidium, licorice, anemarrhena

References

Ahmed, Rauseef. 1987. Tumors Associated with AIDS. *AIDS and Other Manifestations of HIV Infection*. Park Ridge, NJ: Noyes Publications.

Andrews, Carl. 1987. Chinese Herbs in the Treatment of Brain Tumors. *Gateways*, Summer/Fall:2.

Badgley, Laurence. 1986. *Healing AIDS Naturally*. San Bruno, CA: Human Energy Press.

Barton, Keith. 1988. AIDS and Western Medicine. *Proceedings of the Oriental Healing Arts Institute Symposium on AIDS, Immunity and Chinese Medicine*. Long Beach, CA: Oriental Healing Arts Institute.

------. 1988. AIDS Herbal Project. *Proceedings of the Oriental Healing Arts Institute Symposium on AIDS, Immunity and Chinese Medicine*. Long Beach, CA: Oriental Healing Arts Institute.

------. 1988. Current Options: An Overview of Some Treatments for HIV Infection. *Proceedings of the Oriental Healing Arts Institute Symposium on AIDS, Immunity and Chinese Medicine*. Long Beach, CA: Oriental Healing Arts Institute.

Cao, Chunlin. 1983. *Chinese Herbal Pharmaceutics*. Beijing: People's Health Publishers.

Chang, R. Shihman et al. 1988. Inhibition of Growth of Human Immunodeficiency Virus in Vitro by Crude Extracts of Chinese Medicinal Herbs. *Antiviral Research* 9:163-176.

Chen, Dinshan. 1987. *Origination of Chinese Medicine*. Shanghai: Shanghai Traditional Chinese Medical College Publishers, p. 2.

Chen, Meifang. 1989. Traditional Chinese Medicine and Immunology. *Proceedings of the Oriental Healing Arts Institute*

Symposium on Immunity and Chinese Medicine. Long Beach, CA: Oriental Healing Arts Institute.

Chen, Xiangjun et al. 1987. Thirty-Five Cases of Systematic Lupus Erythematosus Treated with the Method of Mainly Nourishing the Liver and Kidney. *Acta Medica Sinica*2(5):32-40.

Cheng, Shide et al. 1982. *Su Wen Zhu Se Wei Sui.* Beijing: People's Health Publications, p. 522.

Chinese Journal of Integrated Traditional and Western Medicine 7(12):711. 1987. Bright Prospects for TCM-WM Treatment of Tumors (editorial).

------5:1:12-16. 1985. Diseases of the Digestive System and the School of Spleen and Stomach (editorial).

Clark, Matt. August 18, 1986. AIDS and the Right to Know. *Newsweek*, 46-47.

------. August 3, 1987. Doctors Fear AIDS, Too: Some Practitioners – Especially Surgeons – Shun People with AIDS. *Newsweek*, 58-59.

Cockerell, Clay J. 1987. Cutaneous Manifestations of AIDS Other Than Kaposi's Sarcoma. *AIDS and Other Manifestations of HIV Infection.* Park Ridge, NJ: Noyes Publications, p. 800.

Cohen, Ann, A. 1987. Psychiatric Aspects of AIDS: A Biopsychosocial Approach. *AIDS and Other Manifestations of HIV Infection.* Park Ridge, NJ: Noyes Publications, p. 580.

Cohen, Misha. 1986. *Acupuncture, AIDS, and Natural Healing:The San Francisco AIDS Alternative Healing Project.* San Francisco: *Quan Yin* Publications.

------. 1988. Paths to Wholeness. *Proceedings of the Oriental Healing Arts Institute Symposium on AIDS, Immunity and Chinese Medicine.* Long Beach, CA: Oriental Healing Arts Institute.

------. 1987. *The San Francisco AIDS Alternative Healing Project.* San Francisco: *Quan Yin* Publications.

Coulis, Paul A. 1988. AIDS Patient Care. *Fourth International AIDS Conference Roundup* 2(5):5-10.

Creemers, Pauline C. et al. 1988. Analysis of Absolute T-Helper Cell Number and Cellular Immune Defects in HIV Antibody Positive and Negative Homosexual Men. *AIDS Research and Human Retroviruses* 4(4):269-278.

Dharmananda, Subhuti. 1988. Antiviral Aspects of Chinese Herbs. *Proceedings of the Oriental Healing Arts Institute Symposium on AIDS, Immunity and Chinese Medicine*. Long Beach, CA: Oriental Healing Arts Institute.

------. Winter 1987/88. Chinese Herbs and the HIV Epidemic. *Practitioner's Guide*. Portland, OR: Institute for Traditional Medicine and Preventive Care.

------. 1986. *Your Nature, Your Health*. Portland, OR: Institute for Traditional Medicine and Preventive Health, p. 2.

Dong, Fangzhong. 1978. In Situ Liver Homeotransplantation. *Shanghai Medicine* 9:1.

Douglas, Paul H., and Pinsky, Laura. 1987. *The Essential AIDS Fact Book*. New York: Pocket Books.

Duncanson, Frederick P. et al. 1987. Tuberculosis in AIDS. *AIDS and Other Manifestations of HIV Infection*. Park Ridge, NJ: Noyes Publications, pp. 530-538.

Fu, Gaoshang et al. 1983. The Effects of Kidney Tonification on IgE and T-Cells of Patients with Bronchial Asthma. *Journal of Chinese Medicine* 5:33-36.

Fu, Qieliang. 1985. Clinical Trial of Treatment of Non-Specific Ulcerate Colonitis by Integreting TCM and Western Medicine. *Chinese Journal of Integrated Traditional and Western Medicine* 5(1):17-19.

Fujimaki, M. et al. 1989. Clinical Efficacy of Two Kinds of Kanpo Medicine on HIV-Infected Patients (abstract reference: W.B.P. 292). *Proceedings of the 5th International Conference on AIDS, Montreal, Quebec, Canada, June 4-9, 1989*, p. 400.

Gallo, Robert, and Montagnier, Luc. 1988. AIDS in 1988. *Scientific American* 259(4):41-51.

Geissman, T A. 1964. Toxicity of *Senecio Scandens*. *Annual Review of Pharmacology* 4:305.

Geng, Changshan et al. 1988. The Effect of Lycium Barbarcem Polysaccharide on H3 Thymidine in Splenic and T-Suppressor Lymphocytesin Mice. *Chinese Traditional and Herbal Drugs*19(7):25-28.

------. 1986. Progress in the Pharmacological Research of the Immunological Effects of *Huang Ji*. *Chinese Journal of Integrated Traditional and Western Medicine* 6(1):6264.

Gupta, Sudhir. 1986. Abnormality of Leu 2+7+ Cells in Acquired Immune Deficiency Syndrome (AIDS), AIDS-Related Complex, and Asymptomatic Homosexuals. *Journal of Clinical Immunology* 6(6):502-509.

Halstead, Bruce W. 1989. Secondary Immune Deficiency Disorders and the Use of Chinese Traditional Herbs in AIDS. *AIDS, Immunity and Chinese Medicine*. Long Beach, CA: Oriental Healing Arts Institute, pp.28-34.

Han, Dewu et al. 1988. Chinese Medicines for the Prevention and Treatment of Viral Hepatitis. *Abstracts of Chinese Medicines* 2(1):105-134.

He, Quanyeng. 1985. The Nature of Lung *Qi* Deficiency. *Chinese Journal of Integrated Traditional and Western Medicine* 5(5):318-320.

Hebert, Rolland. 1989. Western Botanical Medicines and the Immune System: *Hypericum perfoliatum* as an HIV Inhibitor. *Proceedings of the Oriental Healing Arts Institute Symposium on Immunity and Chinese Medicine*. Long Beach, CA: Oriental Healing Arts Institute.

Heyward, Wm. L., and Curran, James W. 1988. The Epidemiology of AIDS in the U.S. *Scientific American* 259(4):72-81.

Hopkins, Kevin R. et al. 1988. The Incidence of HIV Infection in the United States (report #: HI-4066-P). Indianapolis: Hudson Institute.

Hsu, Hong-yen. 1983. *Chin Kuei Yao Lueh: A Chinese Medical Classic.* Long Beach, CA: Oriental Healing Arts Institute.

------. 1986. *Oriental Materia Medica: A Concise Guide.* Long Beach, CA: Oriental Healing Arts Institute.

------. 1989. The Safety of Chinese Herbs. *International Journal of Oriental Medicine* 14(1):5-43.

------. 1988. The Study of Scientific Chinese Herbal Preparation. *Oriental Healing Arts International Bulletin* 13(2):105-125.

------. 1982. *Treating Cancer with Chinese Herbs.* Long Beach, CA: Oriental Healing Arts Institute.

Huang, Hanbing et al. 1982. Systemic Medical Problems of In Situ Liver Homeotransplantation (Report of Five Cases). *Chinese Journal of Organ Transplantation* 1(1):6-8.

Huang, Jigen et al. 1987. The Essence of Kidney Deficiency and the Therapeutic Effects of Kidney Tonics in Elderly Patients with Chronic Bronchitis. *Proceedings of SinoMed '87, International Conference on Traditional Chinese Medicine and Pharmacology.* Shanghai: China Academic Publishers, p. 193.

Hymes, Kenneth B. 1987. Kaposi's Sarcoma in AIDS. *AIDS and Other Manifestations of HIV Infection.* Park Ridge, NJ: Noyes Publications, pp. 747-759.

Ikegami, Nobuko, et al. 1989. Clinical Evaluation of Glycyrrhizin on HIV-Infected Asymptomatic Hemophiliac Patients in Japan (abstract reference #: W.B.P. 298). *Proceedings of the 5th International Conference on AIDS, Montreal, Quebec, Canada, June 4-9, 1989,* p. 401.

Jiang, Shihu et al. 1979. Internal Medical Problems of Liver Homeotransplantation. *Shanghai Medicine* 2(1):1.

Jing, Jinsuan et al. 1987. The Digestive Function of Spleen Deficient Patients. *Proceedings of SinoMed '87, International Conference on Traditional Chinese Medicine and Pharmacology.* Shanghai: China Academic Publishers, p.38.

Klayman, Daniel L. 1985. *Qinhaosu (Artemisinine)*: An Antimalarial Drug from China. *Science* 228:1049-1055.

Klein, Natalie C. et al. 1987. *Mycobacterium Avium*-Intracellular Infections in AIDS. *AIDS and Other Manifestations of HIV Infection.* Park Ridge, NJ: Noyes Publications, pp. 539-547.

Kolata, Gina. February 2, 1988. AIDS Virus, For First Time, is Proved to Infect Colon Cells Directly. *New York Times.*

Krigel, Robert L. et al. 1985. Kaposi's Sarcoma in AIDS. *AIDS: Etiology, Diagnosis, Treatment, and Prevention.* New York: J.B. Lippincott Co., pp. 185-211.

Kuang, Ankuan et al. 1979. Comparison of cAMP and cGMP of Patients With *Yang* and *Yin* Deficiencies. *Journal of Chinese Medicine* 7:21-24.

Kuang, Yuanliang et al. 1988. Study on Lymphocytic Electrophoresis in Spleen *Qi* Deficiency Patients. *Chinese Journal of Integrated Traditional and Western Medicine* 8(2):90-92.

Lapp, Pat Teeling. 1987. U.S. Physicians in Shanghai See New Cancer Treatment Possible. *Gateways*, Summer/Fall:7.

Lebovics, Edward et al. 1987. The Liver in AIDS. *AIDS and Other Manifestations of HIV Infection.* Park Ridge, NJ: Noyes Publications, p.767.

Li, Lin et al. 1983. Treating Viral Myocarditis with Integrated Traditional Chinese and Western Medicine--Forty Cases. *Jie Lin Medicine* 2:26.

------. 1985. Treatment of 100 Cases of Herpes Zoster with *Machixian Jiedu* Decoction. *Journal of Beijing College of Traditional Chinese Medicine* 8(4):15-16.

Li, Zhenghua et al. 1987. The Essence of Deficiency of Spleen and Stomach *Qi*. *Proceedings of SinoMed '87, International Conference on Traditional Chinese Medicine and Pharmacology.* Shanghai: China Academic Publishers, p. 64.

Lian, Yuehua et al. 1987. The Effects of DBH Activity in *Xu Han* (Asthenic Cold) and *Xu Re* (Asthenic Heat) *Zheng*. *Proceedings of SinoMed '87, International Conference on Traditional Chinese Medicine and Pharmacology.* Shanghai: China Academic Publishers, p. 45.

Liao, Wanqing et al. 1982. Treatment for the Fungal Infections in Kidney Homeotransplantation. *Chinese Journal of Organ Transplantation* 3:131.

Lien, Eric J. et al. 1985. *Structure Activity Relationship Analysis of Anticancer Chinese Drugs*. Long Beach, CA: Oriental Healing Arts Institute.

Liu, Dingqing et al. 1986. Two Cases of Lung Candidiasis Cured by Aerosal of Garlic Extract Solution. *Chinese Journal of Integrated Traditional and Western Medicine* 6 (12): 760.

Liu, Fuchung et al. 1985. Correlation Between Trace Elements and Immunological Function in Patients with Vital Energy Deficiency. *Journal of Traditional Chinese Medicine* 26(11):856-857.

------. 1985. Trace Elements and Immunity of *Qi* Deficiency. *Journal of Traditional Chinese Medicine* 11:56-57.

Liu, Jinglan. 1983. Analysis of 102 Cases of Viral Myocarditis Treated by Traditional Chinese Medicine. *Zhejiang Traditional Chinese Medicine Journal* 1:30.

Liu, Xuoshan. 1979. *The Bibliography of Literature of Research Into Chinese Medicine, 1962-1974*. Beijing: Science Publishers, p. 290.

Lou, Jun et al. 1983. Six Cases of Kidney Homeotransplantation *Chinese Journal of Organ Transplantation* 1:33.

Lu, Heshen. 1986. The Immunological Effects of Chinese Herbs. *Chinese Herbs and Immunology: Blood-Regulating Herbs*. Kuanzhou, China: Kuangdong Science and Technology Publishers.

------. 1982. *Chinese Herbs and Immunology: Chinese Tonics*. Kuanzhou, China: Kuangdong Science and Technology Publishers.

Ma, Cuiyu et al. 1988. Combination with Autonomic Function Test to Increase Effectiveness of Chronic Persistent Viral Hepatitis. *Chinese Journal of Integrated Traditional and Western Medicine* 8(12):16.

Mann, Jonathan M. et al. 1988. The International Epidemiology of AIDS. *Scientific American* 249(4):82-89.

Masters, William H. et al. 1988. *Crisis Heterosexual Behavior in the Age of AIDS*. New York: Grove Press.

Masur, Henry et al. 1985. Infectious Complications of AIDS. *AIDS Etiology, Diagnosis, Treatment and Prevention*. New York: J.B. Lippincott Co., pp. 161-184.

Nicholson, Janet K. et al. 1986. T-Cytotoxic/Suppressor Cell Phenotypes in a Group of Asymptomatic Homosexual Men With and Without Exposure to HTLV-III/LAV. *Clinical Immunology and Immunopathology* 40:505-514.

O'Connor, Tom et al. 1987. *Living With AIDS*. San Francisco: Corwin Publishers.

Ono, Katsuhiko, et al. 1989. Inhibition of HIV-Reverse Transcriptase by a Kanpo Medicine, *Sho-Saiko-To* (abstract reference #: M.C.P. 144). *Proceedings of the 5th International Conference on AIDS, Montreal, Quebec, Canada, June 4-9, 1989*, p. 565.

Pan, Xiqing et al. 1988. The Alkaloid of *Viola yedoensis*. *Chinese Traditional and Herbal Drugs* 19(8): 46.

Reichert, Cheryl M. et al. 1985. Pathologic Features of AIDS. *AIDS Etiology, Diagnosis, Treatment, and Prevention*. New York: J.B. Lippincott Co., p. 111.

Safai, Bijan et al. 1985. Malignant Neoplasms in AIDS. *AIDS Etiology, Diagnosis, Treatment, and Prevention*. NY: J.B. Lippincott Co., pp. 213-222.

Shanahan, Tom. 1985. AIDS: Some Facts for the Acupuncturist. *The Journal of Chinese Medicine* 18:11-17.

Shao, Huizheng et al. 1988. The Adjustment of Imbalance of Body Function with *Qi Gong*. *Chinese Journal of Integrated Traditional and Western Medicine* 8(2):76.

Shen, Ziyin et al. 1986. *The Differential Diagnostic Standards of Traditional Chinese Medicine Deficiency Conformations*. Zhenzhou, China: The National Committee on Combining

Traditional Chinese and Western Medicine, Subcommittee on Deficiency and Aging.

------. 1987. Investigation of the Essence of a Symptom Complex. *Proceedings of SinoMed '87, International Conference on Traditional Chinese Medicine and Pharmacology*. Shanghai: China Academic Publishers, pp. 14-17 and 30-35.

Shen, Ziyin, and Wang, Wenjian. 1987. Kidney Deficiency and Aging. *Proceedings of SinoMed '87, International Conference on Traditional Chinese Medicine and Pharmacology*. Shanghai: China Academic Publishers, p. 34.

Shi, Gang et al. 1986. Function of Thyroid Axes of Kidney *Yin* and *Yang* Deficiencies in Patients With Chronic Bronchitis. *Chinese Journal of Integrated Traditional and Western Medicine* 6(3):160-162.

Shi, Lianqing. 1982. Traditional Chinese Medicine's Treatments for Night Sweats. *Modern Medicine and Traditional Chinese Medicine*. Lanzhou, China: Gan-Su People's Publishers, pp. 272-273.

Siegel, Bernie S. 1986. *Love, Medicine & Miracles*. New York: Harper & Row, Publishers.

Situ, Hansun. 1987. Treating Cancer with Chinese Herbs. *Gateways*, Summer/Fall 1987:3.

Smith, Michael. 1988. Chinese Medical Treatment: Frequent Symptom Relief and Some Apparent Long-Term Remissions. *Porceedings of the Oriental Healing Arts Symposium on AIDS, Immunity, and Chinese Medicine*. Long Beach, CA: Oriental Healing Arts Institute, pp. 56-65.

Soave, Rosemary. 1987. Cryptosporidiosis in AIDS. *AIDS and Other Manifestations of HIV Infection*. Park Ridge, NJ: Noyes Publications, pp. 713-735.

Song, Xixiu. 1987. Progress of Immunological Research of Viral Hepatitis. *Chinese Journal of Integrated Traditional and Western Medicine* 7(2):115-118.

Suffredini, Anthony F. et al. 1987. *Pneumocystis Carinii* Infection in AIDS. *AIDS and Other Manifestations of HIV Infection.* Park Ridge, NJ: Noyes Publications, p. 445.

Sun, Qiyuan. 1989. Treating AIDS With the Traditional Chinese Medicine's Treatment Principles for Leukemia. *Modern Drug Weekly of Taiwan.* Nos. 1239-1242, beginning with the May 15, 1989, issue.

Sun, Yan et al. 1987. Observations Concerning a Ten-Year Follow-Up of Cancer Patients Using *Fuzheng* Therapy. *Chinese Journal of Integrated Traditional and Western Medicine* 7(12):712-714.

Wagner, Hildebert. 1985. Immunostimulants from Medicinal Plants. *Advances in Chinese Medicinal Materials Research.* Singapore: World Scientific Publishing Co., p. 159.

Wang, Jianhua et al. 1986. Investigation of Essence of *Xu Zheng* (Deficiency) With Load Tests. *Journal of Chinese Traditional Medicine* 9:59-61.

Wang, Jinyuan et al. 1988. Clinical and Experimental Studies on the Treatment of Leukopenia with *Shengbai* Tablet. *Journal of Traditional Chinese Medicine* 29(1):32-34.

Wang, Xianming. 1984. *Xu Lao and Lao Zhai Differentiation of Traditional Chinese Internal Medicine.* Beijing: People's Health Publishers, pp. 444-459.

Wang, Yusheng et al. 1983. *Pharmacology and Applications of Chinese Materia Medica.* Beijing: People's Health Publishers.

Wong, K. Chimin, and Wu, Lien-Teh. 1977. *History of Chinese Medicine.* Taipei, Taiwan: Southern Materials Center, Inc., P.O. Box 36-22, p. 41.

World Health Organization. 1988. Interview: Jonathan Mann, Director of WHO's AIDS Program, Discusses the International Epidemic. *AIDS Patient Care* 2(3):16.

Wu, Baoji et al. 1982. *Pharmacology of Chinese Materia Medica.* Beijing: People's Health Publishers.

Xia, Xiang et al. 1987. Aging and *Xu Zheng* (Deficiency). *Proceedings of SinoMed '87, International Conference on Traditional Chinese Medicine and Pharmacology.* Shanghai: China Academic Publishers, p. 159.

Xia, Zongqin et al. 1979. The Research of *Xu Zheng* of Traditional Chinese Medicine. *Journal of Traditional Chinese Medicine* 11:2-10.

Yang, Yingzhen et al. 1987. The Effect of Astragalus Membranous Injections on the Heartbeat of Rats Infected With Coxsackie B-2 Virus. *Chinese Medical Journal* 100(7):595-602.

Yang, Zhen, and Ko, Xuefan. 1987. *Yang* Deficiency Causing Exterior Cold and *Yin* Deficiency Causing Interior Heat and Wenger's Autonomic Nervous Types. *Proceedings of Sino-Med '87, International Conference on Traditional Chinese Medicine and Pharmacology.* Shanghai: China Academic Publishers, p. 71.

Yin, Guangyao et al. 1985. The Change of H3-TdR Lymphocyte and cAMP in Chronic Spleen Deficiency. *Chinese Journal of Integrated Traditional and Western Medicine* 5(11):671-673.

Yu, Juan et al. 1988. Clinical Observation of AIDS Treated with Traditional Chinese Medicine. *Chinese Journal of Integrated Traditional and Western Medicine* 8(2):71-73.

Zhang, Daizhao. 1988. Prevention and Treatment of Side Effects of Radiotherapies and Chemotherapies of Cancer with Traditional Chinese Medicine. *Chinese Journal of Integrated Traditional and Western Medicine* 8(2):114-116.

Zhang, Huichuan et al. 1985. Observation of Therapeutic Effects of *Qing-Re-Jie-Du-Tang* on Pneumonia. *Chinese Journal of Integrated Traditional and Western Medicine* 5(9):537-539.

Zhang, Jiaqing et al. 1987. The Acceptor of Adrenic Hormone of White Blood Cells of *Yang* Deficient Patients. *Proceedings of SinoMed '87, International Conference on Traditional Chinese Medicine and Pharmacology,* p. 41.

Zhang, Qingcai. 1988. Clinical Trials of Traditional Chinese Medical Treatment for AIDS. *Proceedings of the Oriental Healing Arts Symposium on AIDS, Immunity and Chinese Medicine*.Long Beach, CA: Oriental Healing Arts Institute, pp. 66-91.

------. 1988. The Traditional Chinese Medicine Rule of Treatment: "Activating Blood and Dissolving Stasis" and Chronic Locomotor Pain. *Oriental Healing Arts International Bulletin* 13(2):141-147.

------. 1989. Three Therapeutic Approaches of Traditional Chinese Medicine Treatment for AIDS. *Proceedings of the Chinese Medical Academy Annual Conference, July 15-16, 1989, at the University of So. CA., Los Angeles.*

Zhang, Yuexuan et al. 1983. The Essence of Spleen Deficiency. *Journal of Traditional Chinese Medicine* 24(8):72-74.

Zheng, Rong Rong. 1987. *Qi Gong* for Cancer. *Gateways,* Summer/Fall:5.

Zheng, Zemin et al. 1984. Treatment of Fifty-One Cases of Herpes Zoster. *Fujian Journal of Traditional Chinese Medicine* 15(6):29-30.

Zhou, Jichang et al. 1987. Treatment of Chemotherapy-Induced Leukopenia with Ginsenosides. *Cancer Research on Prevention and Treatment* 14(3):149-150.

Zhou, Jinghuang et al. 1986. *Pharmacology of Chinese Medicine*. Shanghai: Shanghai Science and Technology Publishers, pp. 289-305.

Zhou, Yong et al. 1985. The Immuno-Regulating Effects of Qi Tonics in Mice. *Journal of Traditional Chinese Medicine* 6:67-68.

Glossary

acupressure--the application of fingertip pressure to specific acupuncture points on the skin for therapeutic reasons.

acupuncture--a natural means of stimulation by piercing specific body locations with needles.

aural and olfactory observation--see *wen zhen* (聞診).

blood--see *xue*.

blood stagnancy/blood stasis--a condition usually associated with long-term chronic diseases, which is due to an accumulation of blood in the veins, the impeded flow of blood through the veins, hemorrhaging, or blood clots and can evidence the clinical manifestations of a dark red tongue, tendency to bruise easily, intermittent pulse, localized pain, tumors, menstrual disorders, numbness in the hands and feet, and dry, rough skin.

bu-yi--tonifying; reinforcing and nourishing deficiencies of *qi, yang*, and blood so as to treat various deficiency symptom complexes.

channels and collaterals--the meridian system of specific conduits for the circulation of blood and *qi* throughout the body, the channels of which are the main conduits and are situated deeply, and the collaterals of which form the superficial network interconnecting the channels and all portions of the body.

cold--(1) the pathogenic cold factor. (2) the cold syndrome.

collapse of *qi*--see *tao qi*.

conformation--see *zheng*.

confusing the heart openings--see *tan-mi-xin-qiao*.

dampness--(1) a pathogenic factor. (2) the dampness syndrome.

dampness-heat--(1) dampness combined with heat as a pathogenic factor. (2) dampness-heat syndrome, a febrile disease characterized by fever, headaches, a feeling of heaviness, body aches, epigastric distention, anorexia, low output of dark-colored urine, and a greasy, yellow tongue coating. (3) other diseases caused by dampness-heat, such as dampness-heat jaundice, dampness-heat dysentery, and dampness-heat leukorrhea.

dampness-heat blended to the lower energizer (downward flow of dampness-heat)--pathologic changes caused by the downward flow of pathogenic dampness-heat into the lower energizer, chiefly manifested as diarrhea, dysentery, stranguria with turbid discharge, and leukorrhagia (see also **lower energizer**).

da tu wen--(1) mumps. (2) an epidemic disease due to seasonal wind-warm pathogens and characterized by flushed, swollen face and sore throat.

debilitating heat steaming from the bones--see *gu zheng lao re*.

defense *qi*--see *wei qi*.

deficiency--a term juxtaposed with "excess" and associated with *yin*; deficiency conditions are generally characterized by insufficient *qi*, blood, or other substances, or by decreased activity of any of the *yin* or *yang* aspects of the organs.

dong gong--a *qi gong* exercise with body movements.

dong wen (winter-warm syndrome)--influenza due to un-seasonably warm winter weather.

dryness--(1) the pathogenic dry factor. (2) the dry syndrome.

excess--a term juxtaposed with "deficiency" and associated with *yang*; excess conditions generally occur when an external evil attacks the body, when some bodily function is hyperactive, or when an obstruction causes an inappropriate accumulation of *qi* or blood.

exterior (or external)--associated with *yang*, this term has less to do with physical location than with the ultimate life significance of an organ; exterior disharmonies are characterized by an acute illness with a sudden onset, chills, fever, and head or body aches.

external evils--pathogenic factors, such as viral, bacterial, or fungal infections, and adverse weather conditions.

fang song gong--a preliminary form of *qi gong* which relaxes the body and mind and is easy to practice.

fei (lung)----refers not only to the organ itself as the regulator of respiration and the location of the exchange of gases between the inside and outside of the body, but also to the activities of transporting nutrients and regulating metabolism of bodily fluids, and so is closely associated with the skin and hair.

fei lao (lung asthenia)--an asthenic condition characterized by coughing, shortness of breath, fullness of the chest, back pain, chills, and lassitude, and due to damaged lung *qi*.

fei qi (lung *qi*)--(1) that which controls the functional activities of the lungs. (2) respiratory air.

fire--(1) the pathogenic fire factor. (2) the fire (heat) syndrome of febrile diseases. (3) the motive force of life; physiological fire (heat). (4) another name for the *yang* principle of certain viscera, e.g., the heart *yang* may also be called heart fire.

five solid organs--see *zang.*

fong wen (wind-warm syndrome)--influenza occurring in the spring and winter.

four examinations--a determination of a patient's *zheng* through an analysis of symptoms in accordance with the principles of a visual observation, an aural and olfactory observation, a questioning of the patient, and palpation.

fu wen (seasonal evil-heat disease)--any acute febrile disease with a prolonged dormancy after the pathogenic heat factor has entered the body, occurring at any time during the year and characterized by the symptom complex of internal heat at the onset.

fuzheng--supporting the body's natural order; enhancing immunity.

gan (liver)--refers not only to the organ itself, but to its functions of storing and regulating blood, aiding digestion, and transporting nutrients, as well as some functions of the central nervous and motor systems and the physiological functions of the eyes.

gan lao (liver asthenia)--one of the *wu lao* (five asthenic diseases) which causes damage to liver *qi* through mental excitement, and is characterized by anxiety, blurred vision, pain in the chest and hypochondrium, flaccid muscles and tendons, and difficulty in movement.

gong fu--see *kung fu.*

gu ji (bone exhaustion)--one of the six exhaustions (*lu ji*); a deficient condition characterized by loss of teeth and debility in the feet.

gu zheng lao re (debilitating heat steaming from the bone) --fever due to a *yin* deficiency, as if the heat were spreading from the inside of the bones to the surface of the skin, usually accompanied by night sweating and frequently seen in pulmonary tuberculosis.

heart--see *xin.*

heart asthenia--see *xin lao.*

heat--(1) although often used interchangeably with "fire," this term is generally associated with external influences, while the latter is associated with internal. (2) a *yang* phenomenon usually accompanied by high fever, red complexion, red eyes, and dark-red urine.

heat in the five centers--see *wu xin fan re.*

he-jie--therapeutic harmonizing, through the use of herbs, to eliminate pathogenic factors.

hot--descriptive of a *yang* or excess disharmony.

huang dan--jaundice.

huo-xue--activating the circulation of blood.

interior (or internal)--associated with *yin*, this term has less to do with physical location than with the ultimate life significance of an organ; interior disharmonies are often associated with chronic conditions.

intestines--two of the six hollow organs, namely, the small and large intestines, the former of which further separates ingested food and fluids received from the stomach into "pure" substances, which proceed to the spleen, and "turbid," which move to the large intestine, where water is extracted from the wastes and wastes are eliminated.

je huang--acute jaundice.

jing (essence or vital essence)--the substance most closely associated with life itself; that which the entire body and all its organs require in order to thrive.

jing gong--a static form of *qi gong* in which the body does not move.

jing ji (exhaustion of vital essence)--one of the six exhaustions (*lu ji*); a deficient condition characterized by blurred vision and hearing impairment.

jin ji (tendon exhaustion)--one of the six exhaustions (*lu ji*); a deficient condition characterized by muscle spasms and convulsions.

kidney--see *shen* (腎).

kidney *yang* (primordial *yang*, kidney fire, congenital fire)-- the functional activities of the kidney, which are the source of body's own internal heat and are related to the ebb and flow of cold and heat throughout the body; when these activities are hypofunctional and accompanied by cold manifestations, the condition is considered a deficiency of kidney *yang* and when these activities are hyperfunctional and accompanied by heat manifestations, the condition is considered an excess of kidney *yang*.

kung fu (*gong fu*)--mastery of a mental and physical achievement through systematic and long-term practice.

lao zhai--consumptive exhaustion; "wasting away."

li qi--infectious evil factors.

liver--see *gan*.

liver asthenia--see *gan lao*.

liver fire--a condition characterized by headaches, dizziness, deafness, conjunctiva, irritability, restlessness, bitter taste in the mouth, dysphoria, and, in severe cases, mania, hematemesis, hemoptysis, epistaxis, a stringy, rapid, and forceful pulse, and a red-edged tongue with a yellowish coating.

lower energizer--the functional segment of the body cavity below the umbilicus and including the kidneys, bladder, and intestines (see also **middle energizer, upper energizer,** and **triple burner**).

lu ji (six exhaustions)--six types of complexes of deficiency symptoms manifested in blood (*xue ji*), vital energy (*qi ji*), vital essence (*jing ji*), tendons (*jin ji*), muscles (*rou ji*), and bones (*gu ji*).

lung--see *fei*.

meridians--the invisible pathways which carry *qi* and blood, and so nourishment and strength, throughout the body and thereby comprise a network which links all fundamental substances and organs (see also **channels and collaterals**).

mian yi--immunity.

middle energizer (middle heater)--the functional segment of the body cavity between the diaphragm and the umbilicus, which includes the liver, stomach, and spleen (see also **lower energizer, upper energizer,** and **triple burner**).

moxibustion--an acupuncture method involving the application of an ignited cone or stick of mugwort over acupuncture points in order to stimulate the body through heat.

palpation--see *qie zhen.*

pi (spleen)--considered by some to be the pancreas, by others to be the spleen itself, and by still others to be the spleen-pancreas complex, but in any case, that which is primarily responsible for the functioning of the digestive system.

pi lao (spleen asthenia)--one of the *wu lao* (five asthenic diseases), an asthenic condition due to overeating or excessive worrying, both of which damage splenetic *qi*, and characterized by muscular atrophy, weakness in the limbs, reduced appetite, abdominal distention, and loose stools.

pi qi--spleen *qi*, which is the post-natal source of vital energy (*zheng qi*).

qi--(1) the nutritive materials which circulate through the body. (2) the functional activities of the viscera and tissues. (3) respiratory gases.

qie zhen (palpation)--one of the four examinations, and often considered the most important; includes feeling the patient's pulse, not in the cursory sense of Western medicine, but in order to determine any disharmonies which may be present in the patient's body; also entails touching elsewhere besides the wrist, particularly at various acupuncture points.

qi gong--a hygienic breathing exercise which uses the mind to guide the movement of vital energy (*yuan qi*) through the body, thereby promoting self-control, concentration, calmness, stability, and the ability to more effectively cope with emotional and health problems.

qi ji (exhaustion of vital energy)--one of the six exhaustions (*lu ji*); a deficient condition characterized by difficulty in breathing.

qing-fei-re--clearing heat from the lung.

qing re jie du--heat-clearing and toxin-eliminating.

qing-xu-re--clearing asthenic heat.

qi qing--the seven emotional reactions which can adversely affect one's health, namely, joy, anger, anxiety, worry, grief, apprehension, and fright.

qi shang (seven impairments, seven *shang*)-- the following causes of undue stress which contribute to the conditions encompassed by the five asthenic diseases (*wu lao*): overeating, which impairs the spleen; excessive anger, which impairs the liver; overworking and prolonged sitting in a damp place, which impair the kidney; exposure to cold-evil and the retention of water, which impair the lungs; worry and anxiety, which impair the heart; exposure to wind, rain, cold, and summer-heat evils, which impairs the constitution; and shock and intemperance, which impair the mind.

questioning diagnosis--see *wen zhen* (問診).

qu-tong--pain-relieving.

quxie--eliminating external evils; reducing the potency of the pathogen; antiviral.

rou ji (muscle exhaustion)--one of the six exhaustions (*lu ji*); a deficient condition characterized by degenerated and atrophied muscles.

ru jing--the serenity which comes from the practice of *qi gong* and is due to the protection of the brain's cortex from environmental stimuli.

seasonal evil-heat disease--see *fu wen.*

seven *shang* (seven impairments)--see *qi shang.*

shan gong--entering the *qi gong* state.

shan han--febrile diseases.

shen (腎) (kidney)--refers not only to the organ itself, but also to some of the genital, urinary, and en-docrinological activities of the body, and is closely re-lated to the respiratory, hemopoietic, and digestive systems, as well as the body's growth, development, and fluid metabolism, and the physiological activities of hearing, and so is called the "root of life."

shen (神) (spirit)--(1) the vitality present in *jing* and *qi*. (2) those aspects of human consciousness associated with an individual's personality and the accompanying abilities to reason, think creatively, and make decisions. (3) the capacity of the mind to form ideas. (4) the will to live.

shen **disturbances**--confusion, disorientation, and/or dementia.

shen lao (kidney asthenia)--one of the *wu lao* (five as-thenic diseases) due to damage of kidney *qi* through excessive sexual activities and characterized by lum-bago, spermatorrhea or disturbances of the menstrual cycle, night sweating, *gu zheng lao re*, tidal fever, and weakness in the extremities.

shen qi--kidney *qi*, the congenital source of vital energy (*zheng qi*).

shu wen (summer heat-warm disease)--any acute febrile disease caused by the summer-heat pathogen and characterized by high fever at the onset, profuse sweating, general malaise, polydipsia, restlessness, and flushed face.

six exhaustions--see *lu ji.*

six hollow organs--the *yang* organs, considered to be not as directly involved with the fundamental substances as are the *yin* organs (five solid organs); the small intestine, large intestine, stomach, gall bladder, bladder, and triple burner.

spirit--see *shen.* (神)

spleen--see *pi.*

spleen asthenia--see *pi lao.*

stagnant water/water stasis--a condition characterized by the retention of water by the body.

stomach--see *wei.*

summer heat-warm disease--see *shu wen.*

tan-mi-xin-qiao (confusing the heart openings)--the impairment of consciousness and mental confusion caused by the invasion of phlegm, including such symptoms as disorientation, coughing with rales, coma, chest discomfort, slippery pulse, and whitish, glossy coating on the tongue.

tan tien--a spot approximately three inches below the navel which is used as a point of mental concentration when doing *qi gong* and other relaxation exercises or meditations.

tao qi (collapse of *qi*)--(1) condition due to the dissipation or exhaustion of *qi* (vital energy). (2) symptoms, such as cold hands and feet, loose stools, and a faint, slow pulse, due to an insubstantial *yang* principle..

Theory of the Five Solid Organs--a fundamental theory of Traditional Chinese Medicine which contends that manifestations of external symptoms reflect the physiological functions and pathological changes of the viscera and that assessments of external symptoms can be utilized to promote general good health and diagnose and treat disease.

triple burner (triple heater)--one of the six hollow organs, the one about which there has been great dispute as to its actuality, though it is generally thought to be one of the following: (1) the entire body cavity, including the chest, abdominal, and pelvic cavities; (2) the lymphatic system; (3) the omentum; and (4) an entity with no location *per se*, but rather the function of regulating water, primarily between the spleen, lungs, and kidneys, but also between the small intestine and the bladder. Currently, the majority of TCM practitioners favor considering the triple burner's functional sections of the body cavity, namely, the upper energizer, middle energizer, and lower energizer, rather than the actual organs located within those sections (see also **lower energizer, middle energizer,** and **upper energizer**).

upper energizer (upper heater)--the segment of the triple burner roughly located above the diaphragm, which includes the heart and lungs (see also **lower energizer, middle energizer,** and **triple burner**).

violent evil-heat disease--see *wen tu.*

visual observation--see *wang zhen.*

vital energy (*zheng qi*, also *yuan qi* and *qi*)--the body's natural ability to defend itself against pathogenic invasion.

vital essence--see *jing*.

wang zhen (visual observation)--one of the four examinations; includes an assessment of the patient's physical appearance, behavior, mannerisms, facial color, tongue, secretions, and excretions.

warm diseases--(1) a general term for all febrile diseases caused by external pathogenic factors. (2) diseases occurring in summer due to excessive external heat.

wei (stomach)--one of the six hollow organs, the one, as in Western medicine, which is responsible for receiving and partially decomposing ingested foods and fluids.

wei qi (defense *qi*)--a part of the *yang* principle which circulates in the superficial, extra-vascular parts of the body and protects the integument and musculature against external pathogenic factors.

wen bing--infectious diseases.

wen tu (violent evil-heat disease)--any acute infection chiefly caused by the heat pathogen and characterized by high fever, headaches, swelling of the head, face, or throat, and hemorrhagic skin rashes.

wen zhen (聞診) (aural and olfactory observation)--one of the four examinations, which includes an assessment of the patient's voice, respiration, and bodily odors.

wen zhen (問診) (questioning diagnosis)--one of the four examinations in which questions are asked of the patient in order to determine the patient's subjective assessment of his/her condition; includes, but is not limited to, determinations of the patient's sensations of hot and cold, perspiration, headaches and dizziness, quality and location of pain, urination and bowel movements, thirst, appetite, and sleep patterns and difficulties, as well as the patient's medical history.

wind--one of the six pernicious influences, associated with movement in the body and usually accompanied by some other pernicious influence or external evil, such as cold or dampness.

wind-warm syndrome--see *fong wen.*

winter-warm syndrome--see *dong wen.*

wu xin fan re (heat in the five centers)--a subjective sensation of heat in the palms, soles, and chest, often associated with kidney *yin* deficiency.

xin (heart)--the organ which provides for the harmonious, unimpeded, and continuous flow of blood through the body, and is also the storehouse for the *shen* (spirit) and the coordinator of some activities of the central nervous system.

xin lao (heart asthenia)--one of the *wu lao* (five asthenic diseases) due to impairment of the flow of blood in the heart and characterized by anxiety, insomnia, palpitation, and unwarranted fear.

xue (blood)--that which is transformed, in the spleen and stomach, from the essential constituents of ingested food, and, using *qi* as its motivating force, circulates in meridians and vessels to nourish the entire body.

xue ji (blood exhaustion)--one of the six exhaustions (*lu ji*); a deficient condition characterized by alopecia and memory loss.

xu han--(1) a morbid condition resulting from a deficiency of *qi* with interior cold, characterized by a pale complexion, loss of appetite, chills, abdominal distention or pain. (2) sweating due to debility.

xu lao--a general debility or consumptive disorder, caused by impairment of *zang* (the five solid organs) and a deficiency of the primordial *zheng qi*, as manifested in the five visceral systems as heart asthenia (*xin lao*), liver asthenia (*gan lao*), spleen asthenia (*pi lao*), lung asthenia (*fei lao*), and kidney asthenia (*shen lao*).

xu re--a fever associated with a deficiency of *yin, yang, qi*, blood, or bodily fluids.

xu sun (also *xu lao*)--deficiency disorders.

xu zheng--asthenic or deficiency illnesses due to insufficient primordial *qi*, weakened resistance to external pathogenic factors, and impaired physiological functions, including deficiencies of blood, *qi, yin,* and *yang*.

yang--as regards its TCM use, a principle complemented by *yin* and generally associated with qualities such as heat, stimulation, movement, activity, excitement, vigor, light, externality, upwardness, outwardness, and increase, and hence with the back of the body and its upper and outer parts, and so with illnesses characterized by strength, forceful movements, heat, and excessive activity.

yie--bodily fluids.

yin--as regards its TCM use, a principle complemented by *yang* and generally associated with qualities such as cold, rest, passivity, darkness, internality, downwardness, inwardness, and decrease, and hence with the front of the body and its lower parts and interior organs, and so with illnesses characterized by weakness, slowness, cold, and lethargy or inactivity.

ying--(1) nutrients derived from ingested food. (2) blood circulating through the blood vessels. (3) the vessels which carry blood and *qi*.

yuan qi--primordial principle; the fundamental force underlying all of the body's life-sustaining activities.

zang (the five solid organs)--the liver, spleen, heart, lungs, and kidneys (the latter two of which are often singular in TCM use) as tangible, discreet, anatomical material, as in Western medicine, and/or as refers to their functions, relationships, and pathologic processes.

zheng (conformation, symptom complex)--a TCM diagnostic unit which begins with an analysis of symptoms, but also includes an assessment of the cause and nature of the illness, as well as the patient's response to treatment, thereby revealing the total state of the disorder rather than a diagnosis of a specific disease.

zheng qi--(1) primordial energy. (2) a collective term for the body's various means of resisting disease.

zhi-dao-han--inhibiting night sweating.

Index